A Political Handbook
for Health Professionals

A Political Handbook for Health Professionals

Marilyn Bagwell, B.S.N., M.A.
Sallee Clements, M.A.

Arizona State University, Tempe

Little, Brown and Company
Boston   Toronto

Library of Congress Cataloging in Publication Data

Bagwell, Marilyn.
  Political handbook for health professionals.

  Includes bibliographies and index.
  1. Medical personnel — United States — Political
activity — Handbooks, manuals, etc.   2. Politics,
Practical — Handbooks, manuals, etc.   I. Clements,
Sallee.   II. Title.   [DNLM: 1. Health Occupations —
United States — handbooks.   2. Legislation — United States
— handbooks.   3. Politics — United States — handbooks.
W 39 B149p]
R727.B27   1985   362.1'042   84-29708
ISBN 0-316-07522-1

Library of Congress Catalog Card No. 84-29708

ISBN 0-316-07522-1

9 8 7 6 5 4 3 2 1

MV

Published simultaneously in Canada
by Little, Brown & Company (Canada) Limited

Printed in the United States of America

The following material is used by permission of NEA-PAC: Table 10.1, Figure 10.4, "Functions and Qualities of An Interview Team," pp. 203–204, and "Interview Guidelines," pp.
204–208.

Preface

As the thousands of books on government and politics indicate, the subjects are vast and the details innumerable. Such a wealth of information tends to overwhelm most persons. They have struggled with units and courses in federal and state politics and government in elementary school, high school, and frequently college or university. In the end, the mass of detail usually slips away from their long-term memory, leaving them with a grayish cloud, labeled "Politics and Government," in some neural trace that is eroding with disuse.

Those persons whose interest, for one reason or another, becomes active usually have become faint of heart when they again encounter the vast array of information and try to stir their dim memories. Because their interest usually connects to a specific area or need, their faintness of heart becomes downright discouragement when they realize that, for what they want to know, the books are neither general enough nor complete enough.

Most health professionals can identify with the description above. Their professions are facing increasing constraint from various laws and judicial precedent. Some constraints are constructive, but others are not. Furthermore, new technology and changes in society's values and needs require health professionals to reevaluate their policies, procedures, and professional goals. Hence, many healthcare professionals recognize the need to become politically active if they are to contribute to the problem solving and decision making for their professions. But where do they start? What do they need to know? We wrote this book to meet that need.

First, we decided to direct a political handbook to *all* healthcare professionals. Our rationale for this decision is the current and projected

vii

growth of the healthcare field, its incorporation of prevention of health problems in addition to treatment of those problems, and the increasing regulation of the policies and procedures of healthcare. This situation requires all healthcare professionals to participate to some degree in political action, not only within their respective disciplines but also in tandem with other disciplines. The "Balkanization" of healthcare action in the political arena will, in the long run, prove self-defeating. Rather than each profession standing alone, a united front will be essential as resources shrink. However, a united front requires a common understanding of political action. This book provides that common understanding of both what something is and how to do it.

Second, the choice of topics and the manner of their presentation has been strongly influenced by our experience in working with a variety of health professionals at workshops, seminars, and conventions. We decided that healthcare professionals would find a general overview and how-to-do-it book useful.

Hence, this book is, above all, a handbook: a compact reference for facts and for instruction. It is a how-to reference for political action. The first step in political action is a general understanding of the forces that at once impel and constrain political action. Unit I, "The Rules of the Game," presents an overview of these forces. Although more than one book has been written on each of the topics, most health professionals do not need a wealth of details when they begin thinking about becoming politically active. They just want a general idea before getting to work. Unit I presents the essential facts. As health professionals gain experience, they can turn to the books in the reading lists accompanying each chapter for the detail they might desire. Chapter 1 defines and describes the four basic kinds of power at work in the political arena, their overlap, and their misuse. Chapter 2 identifies and describes the four kinds of law that shape legislative action and that constrain healthcare professions and professionals. Chapter 3 identifies political boundaries and tells how to discover one's own political boundaries and how to keep track of them. Chapters 4 and 5 focus on the legislature: Chapter 4 describes its composition and identifies sources of power and of information, and Chapter 5 describes the process of legislation and tells how to read a bill.

Unit I describes the overt and covert forces at work in legislatures and enables health professionals to perceive their interaction. Units II and III identify and describe step by step the actions that health professionals and their organizations can take to give themselves a voice in the legislative process.

Unit II, "Politics in Action," presents useful descriptions of negotiating, communicating with legislators, lobbying, and party activity. Chapter 6 defines negotiation, describes its key elements, and identifies the information that a negotiator needs. The art of negotiation is inherent in the activities described in the remaining chapters of the handbook. Chapter 7 identifies channels of communication and describes the process using copious examples. Chapter 8 identifies the two kinds of lobbying, describes the lobbying process, presents a step-by-step description of testifying, and gives a checklist for identifying weaknesses in an argument. Chapter 9 describes the various activities involved in a political campaign. It provides an overall description of a campaign and gives specific descriptions of voter registration and fund raising. The activities described in Unit II will be immediately useful to healthcare professionals.

The actions described in Unit III, "Increasing Political Clout," may or may not be immediately useful. However, they are an essential part of the long-range planning for effective political action, and health professionals need to know how these actions work in order to include them in their plans. Chapter 10 describes networks, coalitions, and political action committees (PACs). Although people in several healthcare professions, most notably nursing, have become skilled in these kinds of political action, many more have not. Often, these people avoid or do not consider these groups because they do not understand how these groups work and what their purposes are. The information in this chapter provides a starting point for organizations wanting to work together for common goals and, ultimately, for improving the healthcare system. Furthermore, some of the step-by-step descriptions, such as interviewing, are applicable to activities described in Unit II. Chapter 11 provides descriptions of all aspects of a media campaign. Small organizations will possibly use only some. Large organizations, or those on state and national levels, should try to use them all. The detail in this chapter should be sufficient to encourage health professionals to use this frequently overlooked resource.

Finally, the Appendices provide names, addresses, and telephone numbers of federal and state offices and of organizations that can provide information. Although some of the federal resources might seem unrelated to politics, the contents of a specific bill or the operation of an organization 'might require the information these agencies can offer. The list of health organizations might seem unnecessary in that most health professionals know their own organizations. However, the listing provides a starting point for information about other health professions and for potential development of networks and coalitions.

We hope that the overviews of the political process and step-by-step descriptions of political activity will encourage more health professionals to become politically active, even if the activity is knowledgeable voting or two hours of addressing envelopes. Even the smallest activity is an essential one. We hope that all readers, whether experienced or inexperienced, will be able to initiate individual action, to initiate and participate in group action, or to expand the political activities and increase the effectiveness of their professional organizations.

We wish to acknowledge Senator Anne Lindeman, Jay Goodfarb, Jules Klagge, N-CAP, NEA, and AEA who willingly shared their political expertise with us. We also gratefully acknowledge Don Gilliland, who gave his time and expertise to prepare maps for the process of publication.

Above all, we thank our families for their assistance, patience, endurance, and humor.

Marilyn Bagwell
Sallee Clements
Tempe, 1985

Foreword

by Congresswoman Geraldine A. Ferraro

The growing importance of health care in this country—together with the continuing need to improve our healthcare delivery system—provides the backdrop for this very useful "how-to" handbook on political action for healthcare professionals.

Authors Marilyn Bagwell and Sallee Clements present an excellent—and easily readable—overview of the political arena together with a step-by-step description of how to become politically active. The book provides both the encouragement and the essential tools to enable more health professionals to become politically involved.

Why the need for such a book?

Health affects us all. The expansion of the healthcare field—and its increased regulation—requires that nurses and other health professionals understand the decision-making processes that affect our healthcare delivery system.

More than simply telling us what political action is, the book gives us the means to accomplish it. Most of us vote, but often voting is simply not enough. If we care about the issues—and about the health of our family and our community—then we must do more.

The book clearly sets forth the means for exercising the range of political actions, from letter writing to grass roots organizing, and the use of media to influence the passage of legislation.

Taking on the "powers that be" is never easy Working together to achieve political power becomes the essential means for producing effective results. Only if we get involved—either individually or in group action—can we expect to be heard.

Blazing new trails is hard. I know, I've done it. As a wife, mother, teacher, lawyer, and elected official, I've worked hard at each step of my career to make a difference. Being active and involved in my community as a parent, educator, assistant district attorney, and member of Congress required a commitment on my part—just as your involvement will require a commitment from you. But the rewards that come from being involved—and making a difference—are great.

Change can only come about if you actively pursue the course for change. *A Political Handbook for Health Professionals* has these basic tenets as its underlying themes: people can participate at all levels of political activity; ability, knowledge, and expertise can counter gender; and, to be effective, the democratic process needs participants from all occupations, professions, and lifestyles.

Healthcare professionals, including nurses, physical therapists, pharmacists and dieticians—male and female—need to join together as a political force because of the increasing importance and need for quality health care in this country.

This extremely helpful handbook will not only get you started in the right direction, but contains the essential elements to insure success as you venture into the political arena.

Contents

A Political Handbook
for Health Professionals

Unit I
Politics: The Rules of the Game

O ne can view politics as a game. It can be exhilarating, frustrating, confusing, exhausting. But as in any game, players must know the rules to achieve a goal. Healthcare professionals will have difficulty playing the game if they have only a hazy awareness that some people have power and others do not, that the action involves lawmaking, that certain boundaries constrain the players, that the legislative players have their own hierarchy, or that the process can be hedged about with more rules and strewn with pitfalls. Such haziness has several drawbacks. First, it keeps many health professionals from trying to play: The whole thing seems too arcane. Second, those who try despite their haziness fumble the ball more than they expect and, sometimes, more than they are aware. They often become frustrated and cynical. Some quit playing. Third, those who continue playing — even those who are not hazy about the fundamentals — get tired, even burnt out.

Hence, playing the political game without knowing the fundamentals is like trying to play an entire season without substitutes, support personnel, or ideas for modifying the game plan if necessary. Furthermore, some people try playing without a full team; they discover too late that they have inadequate resources, have picked the wrong coaches, execute plays that go nowhere, or, worst of all, are on the wrong field, playing soccer when they should be playing football. A knowledgeable coach would, at this point, order the players to go back to the basics: working on fundamentals until they become second nature. Then the players will execute well, avoid penalties, spot the open player and the hole in the opposing line, gain yardage — and score.

To play the political game, then, an understanding of bits and pieces — the isolated plays — is not enough. Unless healthcare professionals thoroughly understand how specific activities such as contacting a legislator or working a voter registration drive interlock with power, law, boundaries, and the legislative structure and process, they will have difficulty seeing how their professional interests interlock with political reality. And the political reality for at least the next decade is the increasing politicization of health care, the wide range of issues beyond health care, and the increasing number of special-interest groups concerning themselves with healthcare issues. The more players who clamor to play, who want to win a share of the political scores, the more imperative it becomes for healthcare professionals to be competent players. They must perceive that their professional interests are no longer separate from legislative interests and that those legislative interests are part of a broad political spectrum. Healthcare professionals need this perception if they are to delineate convincingly why legislators, groups, and individuals should support their endeavors and to describe how they can do so.

In short, healthcare professionals need to understand, *to know*, the fundamentals as well as if not better than the legislators and other players do. The chapters in this unit provide those fundamentals simply and directly. Although each topic has prompted more than one book, such vast detail often obscures the underlying structure. The succinctness of the following chapters will let you see the structure clearly so that you can perceive the relationships among the topics and have a clear, integrated foundation for your political understanding and activities. From such integration comes effective political action.

Chapter 1

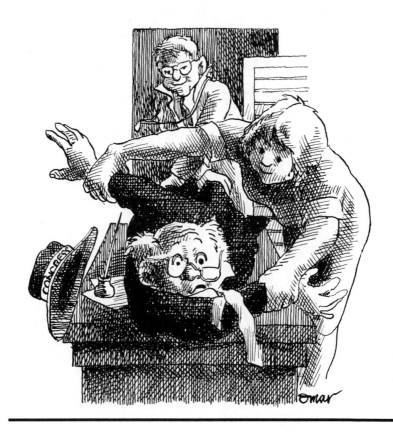

Power in the Political Arena

Effective political action for healthcare professionals rests, ultimately, on understanding the nature of power, its structure, and its impact. Several definitions of power exist, but the generally accepted definition is the ability to influence the behavior of other people. Political power involves the ability to align legislators, individuals, and groups with a particular political stance and to motivate them to achieve through action a desired political result. Hence, in the political arena, healthcare professionals need power to achieve passage, modification, or defeat of particular pieces of legislation that affect the improvement of their professions and of health care.

But using power in the political arena involves conflict. Individuals and groups compete as they try to gain power and to use it effectively to promote and protect their vested interests. Success depends on effective use of power.

To use power effectively to achieve political ends requires an understanding of the kinds of power and of their impact. Like definitions of power, kinds of power proliferate, inviting labels and descriptors that frequently overlap. In the literature on power, identical terms sometimes have different denotations, and similar denotations sometimes have different identifying terms. Furthermore, some classifications contain numerous categories, and others contain few. Some classifications place kinds of power within the concept of power whereas others identify power as a characteristic of leadership or authority. That these differences exist is understandable because such overlap too often creates ambiguity.

However, the purpose for a classification should shape the classification of a concept and the identification of its components. To clarify political power, we have synthesized our first-hand experience with common patterns of classification in the literature in order to provide information supporting a specific end: effective political activity. Consequently, our classification identifies the kinds of power at work in the political arena and the characteristics of each kind. Examples of the kinds of power, the impact of each kind, and some implications of using this knowledge complete each category. The categories are consequently few and broad. In the interest of simplicity, they do not have subcategories; however, synonymous terms, where appropriate, accompany the identifying term to aid those readers familiar with one or more other classifications of power.

Kinds of Power

Traditional power consists of an accrual of precedents. The beliefs and customs that have been passed down year after year become the motivators of behavior. The power of tradition, of the way something has *always* been done by the people who have *always* done it, creates a tremendous inertia with which to contend. The people who wield traditional power can often rely on others' following traditional patterns of behavior because the system, the hierarchy, and the prestige are already in place. To influence the thinking and motivate the subsequent actions of people or groups holding traditional power requires (a) knowledge of the workings of the system and of the hierarchical order and (b) consideration of the prestige of the position and of the value that the person holding the position places on such prestige.

The political system has traditional power. The mechanism, whether a legislature, a party organization, or a campaign committee, has a traditional hierarchy. The policies, procedures, and often some of the people have been in place for years. Consequently, knowing the particular traditions with which you are going to deal is essential. Legislative use of the law; interaction within legislatures and among legislators; initiation of a piece of legislation and direction to its legislative conclusion; various means of informing legislatures and influencing legislation: All of these political actions occur within a framework of traditional power. The following chapters of this handbook delineate the political use of traditional power. For the moment, however, you need to recognize (a) that various political groups encompass specific and general purposes, duties, and responsibilities and (b) that successful use of such groups depends on your understanding of and respect for their traditional power.

You must also recognize that the system of healthcare delivery has, over the last 50 years, *also* become a traditional system wielding traditional power. Legislators, their staffs, and the administrative staffs of legislatures, like the average citizen, are not overly knowledgeable about health, illness, and healthcare delivery (except, of course, those few who have devoted considerable time and effort to learning about them). If one has a problem, one goes to the doctor. If necessary, one sees a specialist or goes to the hospital. Despite the proliferation of popular articles on health, illness, and treatment, the hospital is, to most people, a place where one's doctor can provide one with the needed treatment and care. Tradition, mechanism, and hierarchy are in place to do so. The details of this process are all too often nebulous, both to patients and to legislators. Hence, the traditional power that this system wields is tremendous. Lack of knowledge on the part of the general public and many legislators encourages legislators to rely on the data and arguments that the traditional system supports.

The strength of the inertia that maintains traditional power makes change or successful opposition difficult to achieve. Such achievement requires a thorough identification of the existing situation, the aspects needing change, and the probable objections to such change. Presentation of a desired change should include detailed information that (a) establishes the detriments of the existing situation, (b) describes the change along with its benefits, and (c) anticipates objections and refutes them or demonstrates that the objections are inconsequential or less important than the benefits deriving from the desired change.

Delegated power, or legitimate power, is the power that a person or an organization confers on an individual. Legislators often confer on their aides or secretaries the power to sift and sort incoming information and requests. The amount of power so delegated may range from sorting to summarizing the resulting data to evaluating what the legislator needs to know or handle.

Such delegated power in the offices of state legislators generally varies. Through a telephone conversation you can frequently determine whether the person to whom you are speaking has been delegated the power of evaluating what will reach a legislator's desk. The certainty with which the person speaks is generally your clue that this person has such power. For example, after you state the purpose of your call, the person answering the telephone might suggest (or transfer your call to an aide or secretary who suggests) that the legislator is not actively involved in the piece of legislation at this time but would consider written data delineating the effect of the bill on consumers. From this statement, you can infer that the speaker is also stating the best method of getting your views to the legislator: Write, cite facts, and tie your facts to effects on consumers. If you demand to speak to the legislator, you refuse to acknowledge the delegated power and thereby reject the traditional hierarchy in the legislator's office. By so doing, you jeopardize goodwill and receptiveness to your views.

At the national level, a hierarchy of aides and secretaries is responsible for specific aspects of handling incoming information and requests. The person holding delegated power to evaluate is usually the national legislator's chief administrative assistant.

The legislature delegates power to various agencies to oversee various aspects of its functioning. For example, through statutory law (described in Chapter 2) a state legislature can establish administrative agencies such as the Board of Pharmacists, the Board of Nursing, and so forth. On the national level, statutory law has established the Department of Health and Human Services. The creation of such agencies is, in effect, delegation of power to administer the specified area of activity. Within the legislatures themselves, individuals have delegated power to dispense information, to order agendas, and so forth. The effective operation of legislatures depends on such delegated power.

In general, delegated power within the legislature and other organizations gains strength through an underlying traditional power. Specifically, power delegated through appointment to or employment for a hierarchical position within a legislature, legislator's office, or other group holding traditional power entails duties and responsibilities that are well established and that a job description or its equivalent will usually delineate. People holding such positions can rely on established patterns of operation and general acceptance of their statements and actions. People holding newly delegated power or delegated power within an organization not having traditional power must work hard to establish such patterns and acceptance.

Invested power is power that people or groups consciously give other people or groups to represent or act for them. For example, members of a health profession may give their state and national associations the power to represent and act for them in the belief that the hierarchy of these associations will look out for and act in their members' best interest. Hence, the rank-and-file membership of an association invests power for setting standards and for lobbying for or against legislation. Such invested power derives from the giver's trust: The giver believes that the recipient of invested power will meet specific or general needs.

Should the recipient fail to meet these needs, the giver will usually withdraw the invested power, for example, by canceling membership or leaving the profession. Hence, invested power depends on reciprocity for its continuance.

Voters have invested power in their legislators by electing them to office, and legislators are continually aware that their constituents can withdraw this trust at any time. If legislators suspect that a bill has the potential for strong rejection, they generally consider aligning themselves with the potential majority. However, you need to be aware that legislators may in turn have already invested their power in a person or organization that opposes your stance. Such a situation requires identifying the recipient and what the recipient is reciprocating in order to neutralize the reciprocity or offer something better.

For example, legislators through lack of knowledge might invest power in an organization having traditional power. Specifically, legislators might support the position of a hospital association in the belief that the points that this association advocates will be good for the consumer (and legislators are potential consumers) because hospitals have the traditional power to provide facilities and staff for delivery of health care. In other words, the hospital associations have "always" done it; therefore, they know what they are doing, and their advocacy justifies legislative support. To divest such an association of the legislator's invested power, you must provide the legislator with accurate, detailed information objectively and professionally presented (see Chapter 7).

Expert power is conferred on the basis of recognized skills, knowledge, and abilities of persons or groups. In a state senate, for example, the staff director will gain expert power through his or her knowledge of the legislators, their staffs, and the administrative staff of the legislature, as well as constituents, lobbyists, and representatives of organizations. The staff director knows the personalities and expertise of the various persons with whom he or she deals. The staff director can refer you to such resources as a legislator, an aide or secretary, a lobbyist, or another representative of an organization who will provide you with reliable information. He or she can also suggest the best method of presenting your request. Furthermore, the staff director provides similar information to legislators: which lobbyists, representatives of organizations, and constituents can quickly provide reliable, well-presented data.

Recognition of expert power might, then, be a result of a person's first-hand experience, a person's general reputation, or specific reports of others about the person. In the latter two instances, there is a large element of trust that the reputation is accurate or that the people who report are competent to judge. Any faltering of that trust will prompt reevaluation of the expertise.

In establishing your own expert power or that of your organization, present expertise precisely and find that of others. Overstatement of expertise risks disappointment and faltering of trust. Understatement of expertise risks withholding of trust in the first place. Either case jeopardizes your expert power. Furthermore, you need to recognize that other organizations and persons within your organization, other organizations, and the legislature can have their own expert power. The areas of expertise often range from knowledge of subject matter to skills in implementation or in personal relations. Holders of such power may be a secretary, an aide, other persons having delegated authority, a committee member, or an entire committee. All holders of expert power in areas pertinent to your concerns are valuable sources of information and potential allies. Identify these people so that you can tap their expert power to increase your own.

Personal power, or referent power, is held by persons or organizations that serve as role models or are charismatic. Such power derives from competency with the area of expertise, a willingness and ability to communicate information and to listen, an aura of self-confidence and self-esteem, and the support of others. For example, the representatives of various organizations may perceive that one of their number has some success in getting data to a legislator's desk and having that legislator use some of those data. Furthermore, that person is able to listen to the difficulties other representatives are having and to relay information willingly. The person's poise and decorum impart an aura of assurance in being able to accomplish particular aims. Finally, the person is not adverse to helping other representatives achieve their aims. A legislator, also, may perceive that a person is reliable, willingly and effectively shares information, imparts an aura of being able to do a job, and will provide assistance or data objectively to further a legislator's particular project. Such persons are usually sought for guidance of various kinds and for help with decision making. Several such persons within an organization incline other persons or organizations to request advice and help from that organization.

A common denominator for the effectiveness of these kinds of power is communication. Whether traditional, delegated, invested, expert, or personal, all powers increase in proportion to the holder's skill in communication. The ability to convey—clearly, concisely, and cohesively— your thinking, position, knowledge, or enthusiasm inclines your audience to give one or more kinds of power to you.

Overlapping Powers

Having more than one kind of power increases the power of a person or organization. In fact, most people or organizations possess more than one kind. For example, expert power sometimes forms the foundation of and can maintain traditional power. The tradition of hospital care began with the experience of collected expertise in producing improved treatment and care (expert power), which in turn fostered the belief that hospital care was in the best interest of the consumer (invested power). With the increase in the number and size of hospitals came standardized procedures, which in turn through accumulation of precedent fostered the tradition of hospital care, traditional procedures and hierarchies, and traditional power.

Traditional power can also decrease if persons lose faith in the expert power or believe that it is not in their best interest. For example, news stories of incompetence and research revealing that alternative procedures may be better or cheaper than traditional hospital care have caused many people to seek alternative care for some situations. Such cases have undermined the hospitals' expert and invested powers. With more people questioning the quality and necessity of hospital treatment and care, more people are reluctant to put themselves within the power of traditional hospital treatment and care.

Overlap can also affect both delegated and invested power. A person may achieve delegated power as a direct result of expert or personal power. Or a person who has delegated power may invest power in the organization rather than in the profession, thereby alienating professional peers and subordinates. Such a person can be insensitive to the needs and problems of others when solutions conflict with organizational policies and procedures. Such insensitivity fosters withdrawal of the power that peers and subordinates have invested in the organization thereby decreasing effectiveness of delegated power.

It is apparent that kinds of power are not mutually exclusive. Rather, they accumulate and interact. Hence, it is essential that individuals and organizations desirous of effective political activity identify not just one kind of power but several kinds, their degrees of importance, and their various interactions for all people, organizations, and issues involved in a particular piece of legislative action or political concern.

The concept of male power is actually an overlap, an integration of traditional, delegated, invested, expert, and personal powers. Our personal experience and first-hand observations indicate that expert and personal powers can make gender unimportant. Whether male or female, a person can accumulate expert and personal power by presenting a professional manner: professional appearance, knowledgeable discussion that conveys both professional and political expertise, control of tone of voice and body language. Enthusiasm, urgency, even anger must not blind the person to professionalism, decorum, reason, goals, and other people's reactions.

Some male and female legislators are more receptive to dealing with persons of their own gender, but others seem to make little distinction provided that the person is objective and knowledgeable. It is up to you to identify which of the legislators and staff members concerned with an issue or bill belong to which category. If you meet resistance, determine a strategy that will enable you to negotiate and to increase your personal and expert power by aligning yourself with delegated, expert, personal, and traditional power. It is not at all safe to assume that your gender automatically predisposes a legislator to support or oppose your views.

A spectacular example of expert and personal powers countering gender is Geraldine Ferraro's rise to national prominence as the Democratic candidate for vice-president of the United States. Her career illustrates that personal and expert power plus a knowledge of the way power works in the legislative arena can overcome the "gender gap."

According to *Newsweek*[1] and *Time*,[2] Ferraro's personal power derived initially from her energy, her ability to reason, and her ability to set goals. Her first political goal was U.S. representative from Queens, New York. She determined her strategy and had the energy to initiate it: The necessary 5,000 signatures on her nominating petition were obtained primarily from women as Ferraro haunted supermarket parking lots.

Ferraro established her expert power in her campaign. Her knowledge of feminist goals drew women voters. Her experience as a prosecutor for the Queens' district attorney's office fostered her knowledgeable law-and-order platform, one that appealed to a broad segment of the district.

At the outset, Ferraro recognized the need to reach beyond her initial feminist base if she were to achieve her goal. She needed invested power from a cross-section of the constituency to validate her efforts to achieve personal and expert power in the legislative arena.

Upon election to Congress, Ferraro repeated the process. She applied her energy and logical mind to her ability to set goals and determine strategy. She determined that leadership in the Democratic party was essential for representing her constituency. She listened. She asked questions. She learned the rules of the game, the ways to play them, and the channels of power. She became a team player without jeopardizing her personal objectives and worked within the legislative rules and norms (see Chapter 4). As a team player, she spoke when her colleagues needed a woman speaker. She supported the bills of others in return for their support of bills that she favored. In a male-dominated game, she found a powerful, male mentor — the Speaker of the House. In her willingness to do various tasks and favors for others, she accumulated many IOUs. As she collected and cashed in the IOUs, she was elected to the post of secretary of the Democratic caucus. This post allowed her, due to a change in rules, to sit on the Democratic Steering and Policy Committee, a true center of power (see Chapter 4). She then achieved appointment to the Budget Committee, another center of power. With further strategy, she achieved appointment to the platform chair of the 1984 Democratic convention, a position that spotlighted her political skills and her personal and expert power. In short, as *Time* stated, "A Congressional neophyte, she became a quintessential Capitol Hill insider. She has pulled herself up with intelligence, immense drive, directness and engaging freshness — and by carefully playing according to the rules."[3]

Media accounts of Ferraro cite various colleagues and acquaintances whose descriptions of her include such phrases as open-minded, one of the guys, a feminist, feminine, a team player, a political woman, a cloakroom pol, a nuts and bolts politician, and pragmatic. According to *Time*, the latter has at times angered her female colleagues and some feminists, who claim she is not issues-oriented.[4] Others would say that Ferraro can perceive that the sacrifice of an immediate goal can achieve a long-range goal.

In any event, Ferraro's selection as the Democrats' candidate for vice-president has demonstrated that a person who develops personal and expert power can achieve delegated power and accumulate traditional power no matter the gender. By learning the rules and the power structure and by working within those constraints, Ferraro achieved *and* expanded her power in the political arena.

Misuse of Power

In political activity, most persons and organizations try to establish, maintain, and increase their traditional, delegated, expert, and personal power. As with any good, there is usually a bad: the potential misuse of power hovers over every holder of power. Healthcare professionals and their organizations need to be alert to misuse of power not only among the persons and organizations with whom they deal but also among themselves.

Identifying a negative first requires identification of the positive. Positive power is an action, not a state. Positive use of power, then, motivates individuals and organizations to act willingly toward achievement of positive goals. For healthcare professionals, a positive goal would be to improve both treatment and prevention for consumers of health care by supporting measures that directly improve the quality of that care or measures that maintain or improve a profession's ability to deliver quality care. Such motivation to act willingly implies negotiation and compromise.

Unity of a campaign requires that all participants perceive benefit for themselves either directly as a provider of health care and treatment or indirectly as a member of a particular healthcare profession.

On the other hand, misuse of power consists of (a) forcing individuals or organizations to do one's will; (b) maneuvering individuals or organizations without their knowledge, and hence consent, to further one's purposes; or (c) destroying one's competition. Whether the misuser of power has traditional, delegated, invested, expert, or personal power, the common denominator of such exploitation, manipulation, and destruction is the elimination of freedom of choice. The common end is power for power's sake: a state rather than an action. The misuser focuses on the maintenance and increase of power by any means not on the negotiation and compromise necessary to achieve a result generally agreeable and more enduring to all persons and organizations concerned with the issue or bill.

In other words, when persons or organizations misuse power, power and demonstration of power become the goals. One guards one's turf and tries to expand it, without regard for others' well-being. Healthcare professionals and their organizations, legislators and their staffs, and the staff of a legislature can all become enmeshed in an ever-increasing need to demonstrate the extent of their power and to protect and extend their power. Such larger goals as improving the quality of care or the ability to deliver quality care become merely the arenas in which to demonstrate, protect, and extend power.

It is imperative that persons holding power constantly remind themselves that power is not an end in itself but a means to a constructive goal. Two criteria for constructive use of power will help you determine whether you or the people with whom you are dealing on an issue or bill are misusing power:

1. The need for and use of power must derive from a particular political issue or piece of legislation that affects a stated purpose or goal of your organization or your beliefs as a healthcare professional (for example, to improve the quality of health care).
2. The use of power must elicit the *willing participation* of persons and organizations concerned with the issue or piece of legislation.

Summary

Effective political activity requires individual effort within the framework of a group. Although a person can provide data to a legislator and even convince others to do so, such influence is usually minor. Individual healthcare professionals need an organization in order to reach a large number of persons, to provide them with the information they need to be persuasive, to maintain the initial concern and motivation to act, and to provide the aura of traditional power that accrues to a formal organization.

To attract members, an organization needs to persuade people of its expert power, both professional and political. Such persuasion will encourage people to invest their power in the organization. The personal power of members can be effective in testifying to the expert power of the organization. The personal and expert powers of those holding delegated power will further encourage potential members to invest their power in their organization. Such integration of powers will also be effective in attracting the interest of legislators.

In return for its members' or a legislator's investment of power, the organization needs to maintain and increase its political and professional expert power and that of the members and, in turn, of the legislator. It must continually gather, evaluate, and disseminate information. It must make every effort to educate its membership about political systems and processes, the nature of power and arts of negotiation, and the particulars and options pertaining to specific issues and pieces of current or potential legislation. In this way, the organization equips its general membership as well as those holding delegated power to educate legislators, their aides and staffs, and the general public about the expertise and unity of a particular healthcare profession whose members have invested their power in this organization.

Such integration and responsible use of personal, expert, and delegated power will increase invested power. In turn, the integration of these four powers for responsible political activity increases legislators' and the general public's perception of the expert power of the organization and the members of the profession it represents. If the organization and its members can maintain and increase this integration in responsible political activity, over time the aura of traditional power will become fact. The following chapters provide the essential knowledge that will enable individuals and organizations to identify and use the political power of others and to establish, maintain, and increase it for their own political effectiveness.

Notes

[1]"A Team Player," *Newsweek*, July 23, 1984, pp. 22–28.
[2]" 'Just One of the Guys' And Quite a Bit More," *Time*, July 23, 1984, pp. 18–33.
[3]Ibid., p. 18.
[4]Ibid.

Suggestions for Additional Reading

Archer, S. E. Selected concepts fundamental to nurses' political activism. In Archer, S. E., and Goehner, P. A. *Nurses: A political force*, Monterey, CA: Wadsworth, Inc., 1982.

Beneviste, G. *The politics of expertise.* Berkeley, CA: The Glendessary Press, 1972.

Claus, K. E., and Bailey, J. T. *Power and influence in health care: A new approach to leadership.* St. Louis: C. V. Mosby, 1977.

Deloughery, G. L., and Bergre, K. M. *Political dynamics: Impact on nurses and nursing.* St. Louis: C. V. Mosby, 1975.

French, J. R. P., and Raven, B. The bases of social power. In Cartwright, D., and Znader, A. F. (eds.), *Group dynamics*, 2nd. ed. Evanston: Row, Peterson, 1960.

Gibson, J. L., Ivancevich, J. M., and Donnelly, J. H. *Organizations: Behavior, structure, and process.* Dallas: Business Publications, 1979.

Ginzberg, E. Health services, power centers, and decision making. In Knowles, J. H. (ed.), *Doing better and feeling worse: Health in the United States,* New York: W. W. Norton, 1977.

Grissum, M., and Spengler, C. *Woman power and health care.* Boston: Little, Brown and Company, 1976.

Groppinhoff, J. Profile of Congressional Health Legislative Aides. *Mt. Sinai Journal of Medicine*, 1983, *50* (1).

Jacobson, W. D. *Power and interpersonal relations.* Belmont, CA: Wadsworth, Inc., 1972.

Janeway, E. *Powers of the Weak.* New York: Morrow Quill Paperbacks, 1981.

Jordan, C. The power of political activity. In Steveson, K. R. (ed.), *Power and influence: A source book for nurses*, New York: John Wiley and Sons, Inc., 1983.

Kalisch, G. J., and Kalisch, P. A. A discourse on the politics of nursing. *Journal of Nursing Administration*, 1976, 6, 29–34.

Kalisch, G. J., and Kalisch, P. A. *Politics in Nursing*. Philadelphia: Lippincott, 1982.

Krause, E. A. *Power and illness: The political sociology of health and medical care.* New York: Elsevier North-Holland, 1977.

McClelland, D. C. *Power: The inner experience.* New York: Irvington, 1975.

Mechanic, D. Sources of power of lower participants in complex organizations. *Administrative Science Quarterly*, 1962, 7, 349–364.

Miller, B. K., Mansen, T. J., and Lee, H. J. Patient advocacy: Do nurses have the power and authority to act as patient advocates? *Nursing Leadership*, 1983, 6, 56–60.

Raven, B. H. Social influence and power. In Steiner, I. D., and Fishbein, M. (eds.), *Current studies in social psychology*, New York: Holt, Reinhart and Winston, 1965.

Reiff, R. The control of knowledge: The power of helping professions. *Journal of Behavioral Sciences*, 1974, 10, 451–461.

Rogers, C. *On personal power.* Wakefield, MA: Contemporary Publishing, 1977.

Stanford, N. D. Identification and exploration of strategies to develop power for nursing. In *Power: Nursing's challenge for change*, ANA publication # G-135 5M 3/79. Kansas City, MO: American Nurses Association, 1979.

Stevens, K. R. Power as a positive force. In Stevens, K. R. (ed.), *Power and influence: A source book for nurses*, New York: John Wiley and Sons, Inc., 1983.

Chapter 2

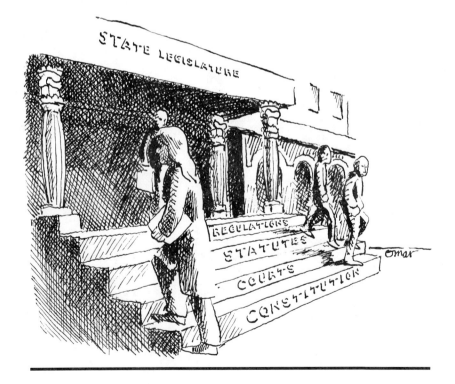

Laws: The Basis of Political Action

Both state and federal governments are assuming increasing responsibility for health care, and governmental agencies are establishing policies and procedures and defining functions of the healthcare agencies, institutions, and professionals. The increasing number of laws concerning health care requires that politically active healthcare professionals understand what law is and who makes it. This understanding is essential if healthcare professionals want to share in the making of policy concerning their professions. At the very least, such knowledge will guide them to the appropriate policy makers or agencies. For example, not knowing whether an issue pertains to statutory or to regulatory law will lessen your expertise in a legislator's mind. Such ignorance will definitely hinder your initial handling of the issue. Hence, this chapter defines *law*, describes the kinds of law and their origins, indicates in general the relationships among the different kinds of law, and suggests places to find copies of various laws. The description of the kinds of law and the indication of relationships provide an overview. The list of additional readings at the end of this chapter provides specific details for specific situations.

Definition of Law

Generally speaking, law is a body of rules that a governing authority establishes and enforces for the orderly conduct of a society. In the United States, these rules of conduct ultimately derive from ancient legal norms (such as Roman law) and societal custom and usage (English common law) that are based on four principles.

According to Fenner,[1] these four principles are justice, change, reasonable and prudent, and rights and responsibilities.

1. *The principle of justice* extends to a person the basic idea of fairness. In essence, this principle acknowledges that one person's actions should not violate another person's rights. From this principle come the guidelines for conduct and the mechanisms for enforcing them.

2. *The principle of change* acknowledges that changes in society and technology prompt changes in the law. For example, society in the last 40 years has increased its expectations for the availability of health care. Consequently, laws are changing to meet this expectation. Some states now permit, within specific guidelines, nurse practitioners to provide primary care. Also, the technology that now permits transplanting a heart or other vital organs has necessitated in many states a legal redefinition of death.

3. *The principle of reasonable and prudent* acknowledges a general standard for evaluating individual action. For example, health professionals who are in similar circumstances, who have similar training and experience, and who are reasonable and prudent would act in a similar manner. There would be common practices nationwide.

4. *The principle of rights and responsibilities* acknowledges that, unless the law revokes them, each person has rights and that certain responsibilities accompany those rights. In other words, a person has basic powers and privileges that obligate that person to specific conduct. For example, the law constrains most health professionals from prescribing medication. It constrains many from accepting clients without a physician's referral. To prescribe medication or treat clients despite these constraints may subject a health professional to charges of irresponsibility and endanger his or her license to practice.

Kinds of Law

The four kinds of law are constitutional, statutory, regulatory, and judicial. Initiative and referendum are often thought of as kinds of law, but they are actually a means of effecting statutory law. This section includes a separate discussion of each of the four kinds of law and of initiative and referendum. Figures 2.1 and 2.2 present a diagram depicting the origin of laws, the relation between federal and state levels, and the hierarchy within levels.

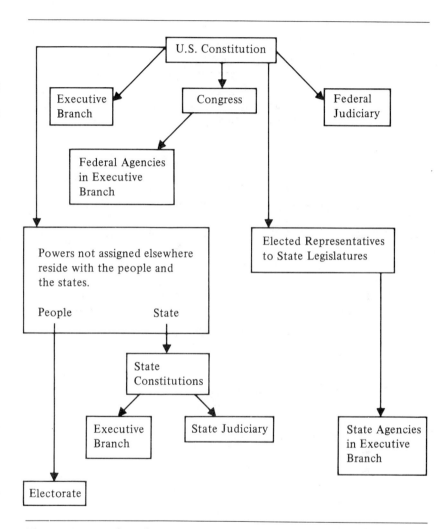

Figure 2.1. *Mandate of Powers*

Constitutional law

The U.S. Constitution established a three-part government consisting of legislative, executive, and judicial branches. It states the powers of each branch and fixes limits to those powers. Hence, Congress must base each of the laws that it enacts on some power that the U.S. Constitution grants.

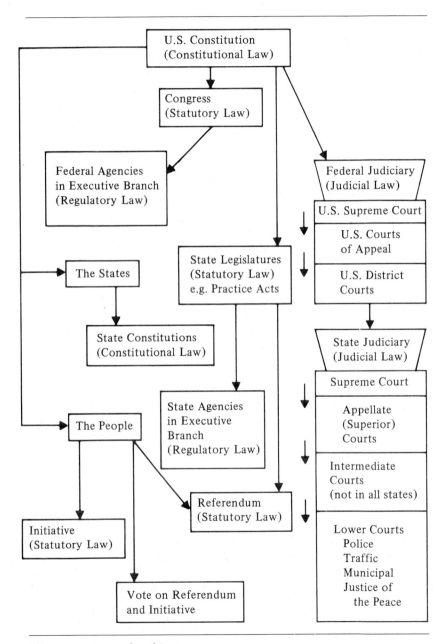

Figure 2.2. *Hierarchy of Law*

The Constitution specifies that those powers not assigned to the federal government reside with the states or the people. However, Article I, Section 8 of the U.S. Constitution states that Congress has the power "To make all laws which shall be necessary and proper for carrying into execution the foregoing powers, and all other powers vested in this Constitution in the government of the United States, or in any department or officer thereof." This sweeping power creates a grey area between state and federal powers and is the source of the continuing disagreement about the boundaries between federal power and states' rights.

The intensity of this disagreement in the early years of the nation (1807) led, in part, to the U.S. Supreme Court's decision that any state law that conflicts with the U.S. Constitution is invalid — even in the state that passed the law. Hence, the U.S. Constitution and, by extension, the laws that the Congress enacts have priority over state law.

As well as assigning residual power to the states and the people, the Constitution also specifies that the states' legislative power must reside in an elected representative body. In other words, to belong to the Union, the states must have a legislative body that is elected by the people to represent the people. This requirement effectively ensures that the states will function by representative democracy, as the federal government does. Hence, all fifty states in their constitutions have established a legislative branch. They have also established executive and judicial branches to enforce and interpret their laws. Consequently, on both national and state levels contemporary law derives from a legislative body (statutory law) and the judiciary (case law).

Statutory law

Statutory laws are broad, general rules enacted into law by a legislative body, whether national or state. Thus, statutory law is also known as legislative law. The purposes for statutory laws are (a) to promote and maintain the state or nation and (b) to protect individual rights, including those of corporations, which the law treats as persons. Only amendment, repeal, or a Supreme Court decision of constitutional invalidity can change statutory laws. On the county or municipal level, legislative enactments are called ordinances or municipal laws.

Statutory law consists of both civil and criminal law. *Civil law* encompasses those legislative enactments that protect individual rights, including those of corporations. Violations of civil law that harm a person or a person's property are broadly delineated in *torts*. Civil law includes such areas as contract law, patent law, corporate law, marriage and divorce laws, and many other areas that concern individual situations not directly threatening the promotion or maintenance of the state.

Those statutes covering areas that directly endanger the orderly conduct of society comprise *criminal law*. This kind of statutory law delineates the conduct that endangers the residents of a municipality, county, state, or nation. Such criminal statutes prohibit conduct and impose penalties for the prohibited conduct.

Although health professionals are indeed affected by such areas of civil law as contract law, the area that affects them daily as health professionals are the statutes that delineate healthcare practice for specific healthcare professions. In broad, general statements, these practice acts can limit what a healthcare professional can do, with whom, how, where, and when. A practice act also establishes an administrative agency to regulate the healthcare profession or assigns the regulation to an existing agency.

Regulatory law

By statute, then, legislative bodies establish and authorize specific agencies to administer to various areas of civil affairs. This type of statute is usually called an enabling act. Because the enabled agencies administer, they exist within the executive branch. There, the agencies define the specific details of their area for administration. In other words, they make the rules, regulations, and decisions that make more specific the general terms of the statute that empowers them. Because these enabling acts authorize the existence and implementation of regulatory agencies, the rules, regulations, and decisions that the agencies make have the full force of law and are known as regulatory, or administrative, law.

The various healthcare boards — such as the board of nursing, the board of physical therapists, an umbrella board encompassing several healthcare professions — all exist under statutory law, as does the Department of Health and Human Services on the national level. The purpose of these regulatory agencies is to regulate various healthcare professions in a manner that protects the individual rights of the public. Hence, regulatory law is civil law. Violations of regulatory law, then, usually come under the area of civil law called torts. If the violation infringes on the promotion and maintenance of the orderly conduct of society, it becomes a criminal offense. However, such classification is unusual. The violation would have to involve intent to harm, gross negligence, or such acts that threaten the orderly conduct of society.

Administrative regulation has the advantage of enabling experts in the field to deal with the problems of a particular health profession; hence, the policies will have long-term continuity. These experts compose the agency rules and regulations that define standards, impose requirements, and generally provide penalties for noncompliance. Usually the rules and regulations are published in proposed form, and there can be opportunity for public hearing or input. In addition, the regulations can be challenged in court if they are enacted without the proper procedure or if their content goes beyond the statutory mandate. The healthcare field exemplifies the extent to which the legislators have mandated by statute the programs and agencies that require a great amount of technical information for their implementation.

Judicial law

Law deriving from decisions of appellate courts and courts of appeal constitute case, or judicial, law. Most of these decisions have, over the years, been codified in statutory law as penal codes, motor vehicle codes, the U.S. Commercial Code, and the like. Although most health professionals have little need in their daily work to keep track of the court system and its decisions, the politically active health professional will find that under-standing how the court system works and the force of its decisions can be helpful in dealing with legislators, in lobbying, in drafting, opposing, or supporting a bill and in other political activities.

The court system is actually two separate systems: state systems, a legacy from colonial times, which are based on the English system, and the federal system, which is constitutionally mandated. Almost no two state systems are alike. Generally, however, they all have a hierarchical system. There are lower, or inferior, courts—tribunals such as police courts, traffic courts, municipal courts, justice of the peace courts, and the like — which handle minor civil and criminal cases. Next are the superior courts, which try most of the major civil and criminal cases. Last are the appellate courts — those courts that hear appeals from the lower courts. Most states have only a supreme court or its equivalent. Some states, such as New York, have an intermediate level of appellate courts between the superior and supreme courts.

The federal system consists of three main levels: district courts, courts of appeals, and Supreme Court. District courts have original jurisdiction (first to hear a case) in most cases of federal law. There are ninety-one district courts, with at least one in each of the fifty states, Washington, D.C., and Puerto Rico. The courts of appeals have jurisdiction over one or more district courts and have ten judicial circuits in the fifty states plus one in Washington, D.C. These courts hear appeals from their respective district courts and have original jurisdiction in cases challenging an order (regulatory law) of a federal regulatory agency, such as the U.S. Department of Health and Human Services. The Supreme Court may review decisions made by the courts of appeal, and it may choose to review a decision of state appellate courts if the decision involves a Constitutional or other federal issue. In addition to these three main levels, there are special courts such as the claims courts and customs courts.

In general, courts attempt for specific cases to make a just rule by considering custom and usage (common law), previous court decisions (precedent), statutory law (including regulatory law), and constitutions. *Common law* may derive from English custom and usage, such as the right of eminent domain, or from more recent custom and usage — that which is customarily done or commonly used throughout a state or the nation. It may, occasionally, derive from a well-argued belief, as the right to privacy evolved from Brandeis's argument published in a law review.

Precedents are court decisions in cases prior to the one being argued. In other words, both trial and appellate courts can use a previous decision as an example, reason, or justification in their proceedings and decisions. These precedents, however, do not have the force of law. Appellate courts and federal courts of appeal can use them as guides or set them aside. Other trial courts can also set them aside. On the other hand, other trial courts can cite them for years, in essence saying, "Everybody knows what

X means. Look at the case of *A vs. B.*" Sometimes tracing these citings of precedents back to the initial precedent can be enlightening or surprising. It may even provide an argument that can weaken the force of the intervening precedents.

The appeal of a decision of a trial court results in a decision from the appellate court or court of appeal that *does* have the force of law for the courts under its jurisdiction. A case possibly having a broad, nationwide application potentially involves federal statutory or case law and might be appealed all the way to the U.S. Supreme Court. The resulting decision will establish, refine, or set aside a federal law and the related state laws within the framework of the values embodied in the Constitution.

In essence, then, case law refines existing statutory law, establishes law where no statute exists, and ensures that constitutional values continue. For example, phrases such as "procedures commensurate with the education and training" are general phrases that court decisions can clarify. Referring to custom and usage as well as to precedent and reviewing the statute and pertinent regulatory laws, all within a constitutional framework, the court determines the rule(s) of conduct in a particular state or in the nation for a reasonable and prudent health professional having a particular kind and amount of training and education.

The courts also concern themselves with establishing law to cover new situations. As new technology develops and as society's values change, the courts will be involved. For example, if a child is a ward of the court and if both the doctors and the parents request that the child, because of his medical problems, be placed on a no-code status, who has the authority to so place the child on a no-code status? So far, two superior courts have decided that they have the right. The first court established six criteria for ruling in favor of a no-code. The second court followed the precedent of the first, and a third superior court is currently hearing a similar case. Hence, the matter is still one of precedent, leaving each court free to decide. Should this current case or a future case reach the appellate court, the decision of that court will then become law for that state or the lower courts within its jurisdiction.

Courts, then, are concerned with the application and interpretation of the law. Because the cases they hear are both civil and criminal, the courts can make both civil and criminal law.

Initiative

Another way to make law is the initiative, a procedure that allows individuals or groups to propose legislation by circulating and signing petitions. There are two kinds of initiative: direct and indirect. Direct initiative places the proposed legislation directly on the ballot. Indirect initiative submits the proposed legislation to the legislative body. If the legislature fails to enact it into law during a specified time, the initiative then goes to the ballot. A telephone call to your department of state (see Appendix A) will tell you whether one or both kinds are used in your state. Use of the initiative has been increasing in recent years when people become dissatisfied with legislative action or inaction.

There are two major problems with this procedure: words and special interest. First, rarely do the persons drafting the initiative carefully weigh the legal impact of the words they use. Hence, should the initiative pass into law, it often results in applications that the initiators and signers did not intend. These unintended applications can cause as many or more difficulties than the intended applications resolve. Second, there is little or no effort to weigh and perhaps accommodate other views. Often the initiative is a means by which a group having a single or special interest can impose its will. Frequently, the signers of such a petition do not fully understand what they are signing.

In essence, then, an initiative can limit representative democracy. On the other hand, a well-drafted initiative that truly reflects a need of the diverse citizenry can serve as a corrective measure.

Referendum

A final means of lawmaking is the referendum, a procedure whereby a state legislative body places proposed legislation on the ballot for the citizens' decision. Some referenda are mandated; that is, some types of legislation, such as constitutional amendments and bond issues, must have the popular vote. Others are optional. In some states, the legislative body can choose to place proposed legislation before the public. In other states, such proposed legislation is set aside to await petitions from the people requesting that the proposed legislation go on the ballot for popular vote. A telephone call to the information desk of your state legislature will inform you which procedure your state legislature uses. Whether mandatory or either kind of optional referendum, a majority of the popular vote enacts the proposal into law.

Health Care and the Law

A current issue in Arizona has involved several methods of law-making and will undoubtedly involve more before the issue reaches resolution.

In the past, state agencies, empowered by the legislature, have regulated several aspects of hospital activity, as for example the determination of numbers of hospitals and of beds. Consumers have become upset about the escalating costs of hospital care, and hospitals have become defensive. Various discussions about putting a lid on costs have occurred among hospital administrators, consumers, agency personnel, and legislators — all with little progress. Consequently, large corporations (who pay a portion or all of their employees' escalating health insurance costs) formed a coalition to urge the legislature to take action. The hospital association lobbied intensely against action. Eventually, both sides initiated bills and lobbied health professionals and their organizations for their support. The corporate coalition proposed sharp restrictions on cost and an agency to regulate the hospitals. The hospital association proposed a flexible scale for costs. Neither bill was enacted.

During the discussion, initiation of bills, and lobbying, the coalition was also circulating petitions for two initiatives. One initiative proposed a constitutional amendment for state regulation of hospitals, and the other proposed a regulatory agency to control hospital construction and rates. After gathering more signatures than the minimum required to place the initiatives on the ballot, the coalition refrained from filing the petitions with the office of the secretary of state. It still hoped to force the legislature to take action.

The governor called a special session of the legislature to deal with the issue. However, despite a nonpartisan effort, no agreement seemed to be forthcoming. At this point, the coalition filed its petitions, the nonpartisan effort dissolved, and the majority party of the legislature countered with three referenda. One proposed, among other items, to limit rate increases to an inflation index through June 30, 1986, and authorized preparations for deregulation. Another proposed a regulatory formula that would become effective January 1, 1986, if the legislature fails to act on deregulation. A third proposed a constitutional amendment for state regulation of rates until 1990—in essence, a sunset bill (which set an expiration date for regulation of rates) for the second referendum aimed for deregulation.

The November 1984 ballot put the forces for regulation—the coalition's initiatives—and those for deregulation—the partisan referenda—to popular vote. However, the voters rejected all five propositions on the ballot, and the issue returned to the legislature. Had any proposition become law, the intensity of the issue would probably have led to a test case in the judicial system. Depending on whether the decision had been appealed and on how far it had been appealed, judicial decision could have not only confirmed or rejected law for Arizona but also provided a decision that other state courts and federal courts could have used as precedent.

To recapitulate: The lack of regulatory authority led to attempts to enact statutory law. Failure to do so led to initiatives and countering referenda, both of which included constitutional amendments. If any one of these had passed, the odds were great that the issue would have wound up in the courts, thereby eliciting judicial law. Because the issue has been cost of care, *all* health professionals in Arizona have been involved to greater or lesser degrees.

Summary

The law affects healthcare professionals in many ways: through constitutions, statutes, regulations, and judicial decisions. Constitutional law generally protects human rights, both clients' rights and healthcare professionals' rights. Statutory laws concern our civil rights and identify those torts and criminal acts that affect us. Statutory law sets forth the practice acts under which we function and establishes the regulatory agencies. These regulatory agencies, our boards, establish the regulatory laws that define standards, impose requirements, and establish penalties for noncompliance. Judicial decisions refine these statutory and regulatory laws, establish laws or precedent where no law exists, ensure our civil rights, and impose penalties if we violate another person's civil rights or commit a criminal act. Since both federal and state governments are increasing their responsibilities in the area of health care, healthcare professionals must understand the kinds of law that underlie the policies, procedures, and functions governing their professions. With such knowledge, they can increase the effectiveness of the political action they find necessary.

Note

[1]K. M. Fenner, *Ethics and Law in Nursing: Professional Perspectives.* New York: D. Van Nostrand Company, 1980, pp. 83–85.

Suggestions for Additional Reading

Annas, G. J., Glantz, L. H., and Katz, B. F. *The rights of doctors, nurses and allied health professionals.* A Discus Book, 1981.

Austin, R. *The governing of men,* 4th ed. Hinsdale, IL: The Dryden Press, 1975.

Conference on legal controversies in nursing. Sponsored by the American Society of Law and Medicine in cooperation with the Colorado Hospital Association and Colorado Nurses Association. Denver, January 17–18, 1980.

Davies, J. *Legislative law and process.* St. Paul, MN: West Publishing Co., 1975.

Dickerson, R. *Legislative drafting.* Westport CT: Greenwood Press, 1977.

Federal Elections, *Code of Federal Regulations,* Office of the Federal Register National Archives and Records Service. General Service Administration, Washington, DC; July, 1983.

Fenner, K. *Ethics and law in nursing: Professional perspectives.* New York: D. Van Nostrand Co., 1980.

Hemelt, M. D., and Mackert, M. E. *Dynamics of law in nursing and health care.* Reston, VA: Reston Publishing Co., 1978.

How Federal laws are made. Washington, DC: Want Publishing Co., 1982.

Kelly, L. Y. *Dimensions of professional nursing,* 4th ed. New York: MacMillan Publishing Co., Inc., 1981.

Rothman, D. A., and Rothman, N. L. *The professional nurse and the law.* Boston: Little, Brown and Company, 1977.

Wing, K. *The law and the public's health.* St. Louis: C. V. Mosby, 1976.

Chapter 3

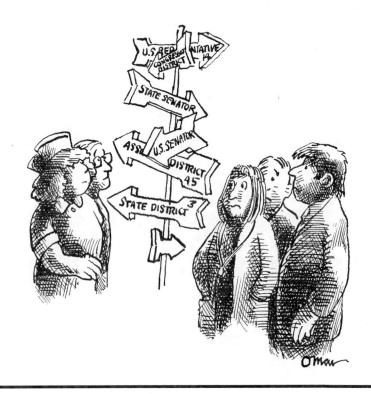

Political Boundaries

Most health professionals must, at one time or another, deal with three or four levels of government: federal, state, county/township/ parish, and municipality. Keeping the boundaries of these political divisions and their subdivisions clear becomes a chore for us because many of these boundaries often differ from geographic boundaries. Also, we don't need to remember them every day. However, political action starts with knowing your political boundaries. Hence, this chapter describes federal, state, and local political boundaries, provides representative maps that demonstrate variations in federal and state boundaries, suggests means of determining the federal, state, and local boundaries of your state, and provides a means of keeping track of them.

Federal Boundaries

Every state has two senators representing it in the U.S. Senate. The boundaries for U.S. Senate are the state boundaries since all voters in a state can vote for both senators, which means.in political terminology that the senators are elected *at large*. Senators are elected for 6 year terms, and the terms are staggered — that is, the two senators do not run for office at the same time.

Through statutory law, Congress has limited the number of U.S. representatives to 435. Judicial law, in the U.S. Supreme Court decision in *Reynolds vs. Sims* (1964), has established the principle of one person, one vote. In other words, the number of persons that each U.S. representative represents must be as nearly equal as possible. The average Congressional

35

district now encompasses approximately 500,000 persons. Because House membership remains at 435, the number that each represents rises or falls according to the distribution of the total U.S. population. If the population of a state, according to the last U.S. census, entitles it to only one U.S. representative, the voters elect the representative at large. Hence, the Congressional boundaries are those of the state. According to the 1980 U.S. census, Alaska, Delaware, North Dakota, South Dakota, Vermont, and Wyoming are entitled to only one U.S. representative. An increase or decrease in population can change the number of U.S. representatives that a state has and necessitate a readjustment of Congressional districts or require the creation or loss of an entire district. States that gain population may elect the new U.S. representative at large until the legislative body of the state can enact changes in district boundaries. Currently, the number of U.S. representatives per state ranges from 1 to 45 (California). U.S. representatives are elected for a 2-year term, and the entire membership of the House of Representatives comes up for election every even-numbered year. Refer to the maps at the end of this chapter for samples of Congressional districts.

To determine your Congressional District for electing a U.S. representative to the U.S. House of Representatives, write or call the office of secretary of state for your state (see Appendix A).

State Boundaries

Legislative branch

The U.S. Constitution mandates that all states have a legislative body, variously known as a legislature, legislative assembly, general assembly, or general court. Like Congress, 49 of these legislative bodies are bicameral, having an upper house (senate) and a lower house (representative, assembly, etc.). Nebraska has a unicameral (one-house) legislative body.

You can determine your state legislative district in several ways. Call your secretary of state's office to request a state legislative map. Or call your county elections office to make the same request. Frequently, you will learn it over the phone. Or call your Democratic or Republican headquarters and give your address. By telephone you will learn your legislative district and precinct. The telephone numbers for these offices are listed in Appendix A.

The number and kind of state legislative districts vary from state to state and may be mandated by state constitution. Some states have separate districts for the two houses of their legislative bodies. Other states have one district for both. The districts might correspond to county lines, or they might differ. See the maps at the end of this chapter, pages 45–57.

The number of legislators elected from each district also varies (see the maps). There is usually one state senator from each district, but there may be more than one state representative from each district. Nebraska elects from each district one state representative to its unicameral legislature. The number of state legislators ranges from 49 (Nebraska) to 424 (New Hampshire). However, no matter how many districts or how many state representatives those districts have, the principle of one person, one vote applies: The number of persons each represents must be as nearly equal as is possible. The length of the term of office also varies from state to state. Some legislators are elected to 2 year terms, some to 4 year terms; see Table 3.1.

Executive branch

The executive branches of state government are also varied. Most states elect the majority of their state officials in statewide general elections (at large). Some, however, use a cabinet system in which a governor elected in a statewide election appoints the other executive members of the state government. Such appointments usually must have the approval of at least one house of the legislative body. Either way, the political boundaries for the executive officials, elected at large, are the geographic boundaries of the state. The important point here is to know whether your state elects its executive officials or whether the governor appoints them. A call to the secretary of state's office in your state can elicit the procedure.

Judicial branch

Variety extends even to the judicial system. Some states elect their judges and justices of the peace; others don't. If elected, some may be elected at large, and some from specified districts, which usually correspond to the legislative districts of the lower house.

If your state elects judges and justices of the peace, get the list and current names of those elected at large and those from your district. A call

Table 3.1. *Terms of Office for State Legislators*

State	Senate Term	House Term	State	Senate Term	House Term
Alabama	4	4	Montana	4[b]	2
Alaska	4	2	Nebraska	4	2
Arizona	2	2	Nevada	4	2
Arkansas	4	2	New Hampshire	2	2
California	4	2	New Jersey	4[c]	2
Colorado	4	2	New Mexico	4	2
Connecticut	2	2	New York	2	2
Delaware	4	2	North Carolina	2	2
Florida	4	2	North Dakota	4	2
Georgia	2	2	Ohio	4	2
Hawaii	4	2	Oklahoma	4	2
Idaho	2	2	Oregon	4	2
Illinois	4[a]	2	Pennsylvania	4	2
Indiana	4	2	Rhode Island	2	2
Iowa	4	2	South Carolina	4	2
Kansas	4	2	South Dakota	2	2
Kentucky	4	2	Tennessee	4	2
Louisiana	4	4	Texas	4	2
Maine	2	2	Utah	4	2
Maryland	4	4	Vermont	2	2
Massachusetts	2	2	Virginia	4	2
Michigan	4	2	Washington	4	2
Minnesota	4	2	West Virginia	4	2
Mississippi	4	4	Wisconsin	4	2
Missouri	4	2	Wyoming	4	2

[a]Every 10 years, beginning with 1972, all senators are up for reelection. The three groups of Senate districts follow different patterns for terms of office: One group elects senators for terms of 4, 4, 2 years; another for terms of 4, 2, 4 years; another for 2, 4, 4 years.
[b]After each decennial reapportionment, lots are drawn for half of the senators to serve an initial 2 year term. Later terms are 4 years.
[c]Senate terms beginning in January of the second year following the U.S. Census are 2-year terms.

to the city or state attorney's office will usually elicit this information. As various decisions come to your attention via newspaper, television, or radio, note on your list the decision. In this way, you will have some recollection of a particular candidate's adequacy, or even a stance for matters pertaining to health care, and can cast a knowledgeable vote.

Local Boundaries

Most municipalities and counties, townships, or parishes elect their officials at large for various terms of office. If your city has districts — a ward system for example — find out what officials are elected from your district and the names of the current office holders. If you know their names, you are more likely to keep track of their positions on various local matters pertaining to health care. A call to the city or town clerk or the county elections office will usually elicit this information. From your address, including zip code, the person answering can determine your district. The county elections office can also tell you the names of your county, township, or parish officials.

Keeping Track

With so many political districts, positions, and names to remember, a master list such as the following can be useful.

Master List of My Political Boundaries and Representatives
   U.S. Senators
   1.
   2.

   Congressional District #2
   1.

   State District #8
   Senate
   1.

   House of Representatives
   1.
   2.

   City — Ward #3
   Councilperson
   Justice of the Peace
   1.
   2.

Judges
   County
   1.
   2.

File this list somewhere handy — an address book, a calendar, or a card for your wallet.

Regulatory Agencies

Officials of regulatory agencies are appointed rather than elected. However, you should be aware of which agencies are federal and which are state so you will know where to direct your questions or political activity. You should also become familiar with the inner workings of the agencies that are important to you. Many of them can be quite complex. Figure 3.1 displays the complex system of the U.S. Department of Health and Human Services.

In addition, the states and, usually, the counties/townships/parishes have their respective departments of health services, often known in abbreviated form as state health departments, county health departments, or the like. The states and their counties vary in their departmental organization. State health departments can usually supply an organizational chart upon request. The counties might or might not be able to do so. If they have none printed, you should take the time to compile one for your county. Your profession's regulatory agency or the state health department might be able to help. You can also make an appointment with a county health official. Explain that you are interested in knowing what departments exist within that county health department and what their lines of authority are. That is, what departments there are, how these departments relate to each other, and who is responsible to whom. Then take notes, asking questions to clarify titles and relationships. Later from your notes, devise a chart that displays the organization. Verify the chart with the official who gave you the information.

Although this research might seem more trouble than it is worth, politically active health professionals realize that having handy such political details as regulatory boundaries will be useful and time-saving at some

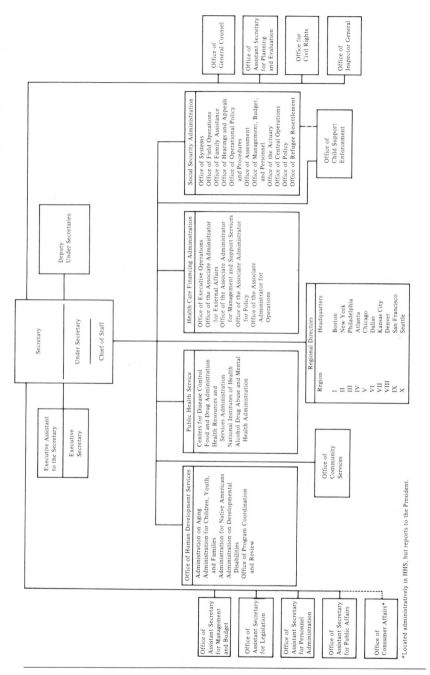

Figure 3.1. *Department of Health and Human Services*

later point. The more political knowledge you have, the more efficient and effective you are.

Summary

Knowing your political boundaries and the names of the U.S. and state legislators, state officials, and state judges elected from your districts is essential for political action. The viewpoints, actions, and decisions of these people can affect the manner in which you are permitted to provide health care, the environment in which you provide it, and even the status of your healthcare profession. You need to know who these people are, what their political views about health care are, and what their decisions have been. Such knowledge can make you an interested and discriminating voter. It can also provide you with a list of resource people who can clarify your questions about law and legislation.

Suggestions for Additional Reading

Growe, J.A. *The Minnesota legislative manual, 1981–82.* St. Paul: State of Minnesota, 1981.

Jacobs, H., and Vines, K. *Politics in the American states: A comparative analysis,* 3rd ed. Boston: Little, Brown and Company, 1976.

The United States government manual, 1981–1982. Washington, DC: U.S. Government Printing Office, 1981.

Wasserman, Gary. *The basics of American politics,* 3rd. ed. Boston: Little, Brown and Company, 1982.

Wiggins, C. *Arizona legislature.* Phoenix, AZ: Arizona Legislature, 1974.

Appendix: Congressional and Legislative Maps

The maps in this section illustrate the variety of Congressional and legislative boundaries. The maps of Congressional boundaries also clearly reveal population centers of the states. The maps of legislative boundaries show the various divisions for senatorial and representative districts, if any, and the variety in the numbers of senators and representatives that districts elect. Such variety demonstrates that you should not assume that one state is like another. This representative selection of maps clearly reveals the diversity.

1. Nebraska has two types of districts.
   - The Congressional District Map shows the boundaries for the three U.S. representatives. It also clearly reveals population centers, the smaller districts being more densely populated.
   - The Legislative District Map shows the 49 boundaries for the election of one nonpartisan state senator from each district to the unicameral legislature.
2. South Dakota also has only two types of districts.
   - The Congressional boundaries are those of the state because South Dakota's population entitles it to only one U.S. representative.
   - The Legislative District Map is representative of those states electing state senators and representatives from the same district. South Dakota elects one state senator and two state representatives from each of its thirty-five districts.
3. Georgia has three types of districts.
   - The Congressional District Map shows the legislative apportionment for the ten U.S. representatives.
   - The Senatorial District Map shows the 56 boundaries for election of one state senator per district.
   - The Representative District Map shows the district boundaries for election of 180 state representatives. The population within these boundaries determines the number of representatives elected from a district (one to five in Georgia).

4. Connecticut
   - The Congressional District Map shows the legislative apportionment for six U.S. representatives.
   - The Senatorial District Map shows the thirty-six boundaries for election of one senator per district.
   - The Assembly District Map shows the boundaries for election of each of Connecticut's 151 representatives.
5. West Virginia
   - The Congressional District Map shows the legislative apportionment for four U.S. representatives.
   - The Senatorial District Map shows boundaries that adhere where possible to county lines. Also, each of the seventeen districts elects two senators.
   - The Delegate District Map clearly shows the boundaries for election of one to twelve state delegates from forty districts.

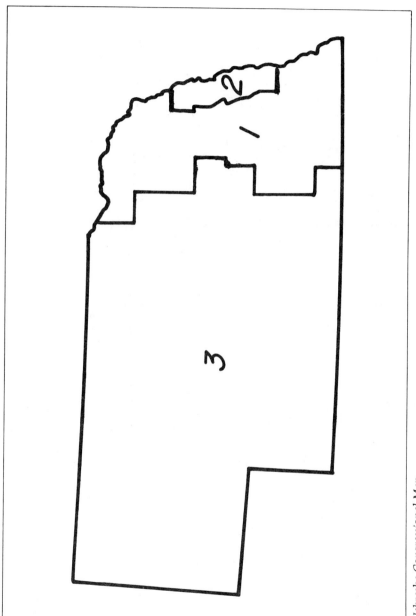

Nebraska Congressional Map

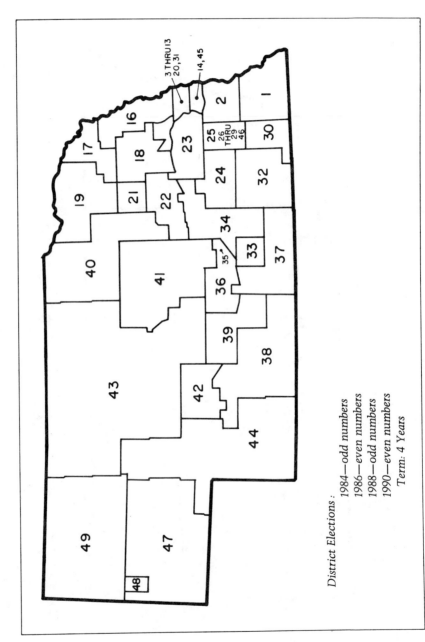

District Elections :

1984—odd numbers
1986—even numbers
1988—odd numbers
1990—even numbers

Term: 4 Years

Nebraska Legislative Map

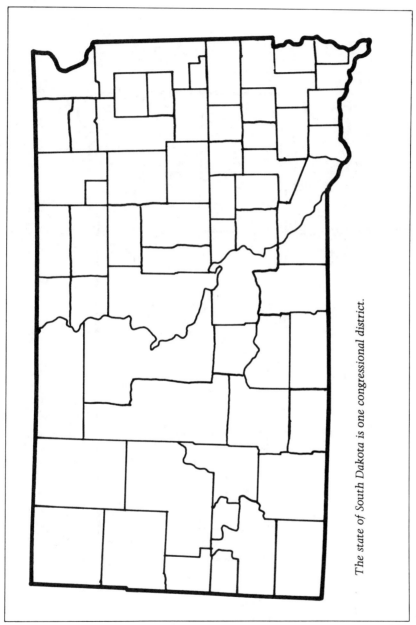

The state of South Dakota is one congressional district.

South Dakota Congressional Map

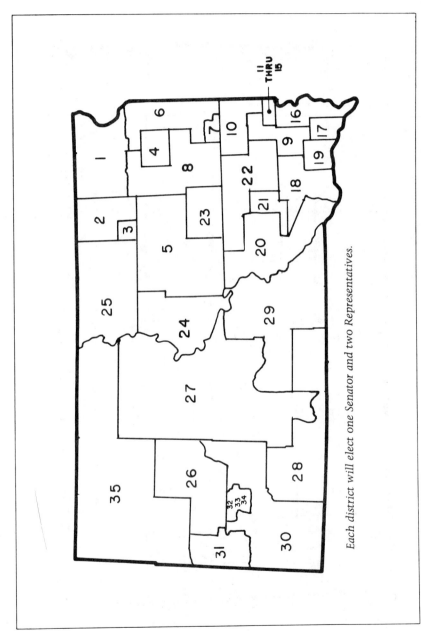

Each district will elect one Senator and two Representatives.

South Dakota Legislative Map

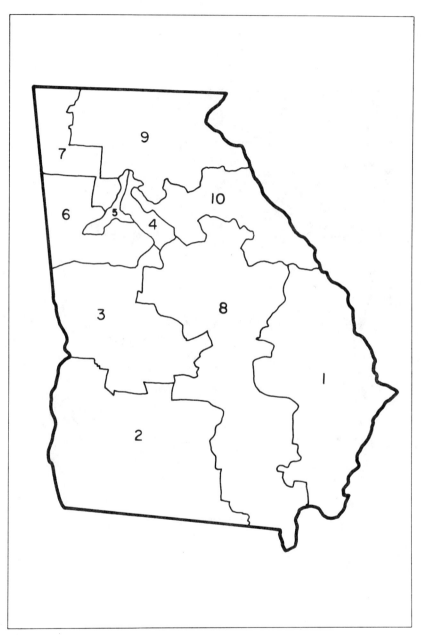

Georgia Congressional Map

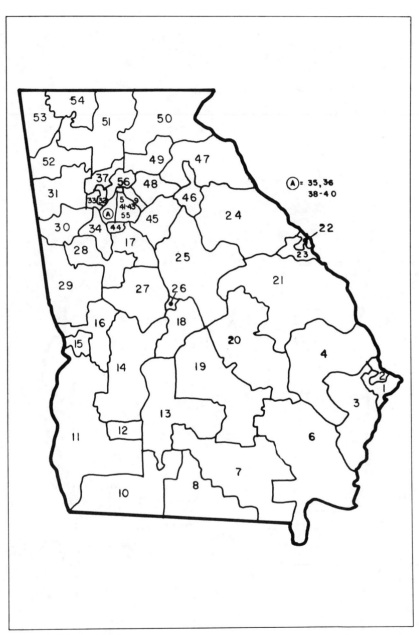

Georgia Senatorial Map

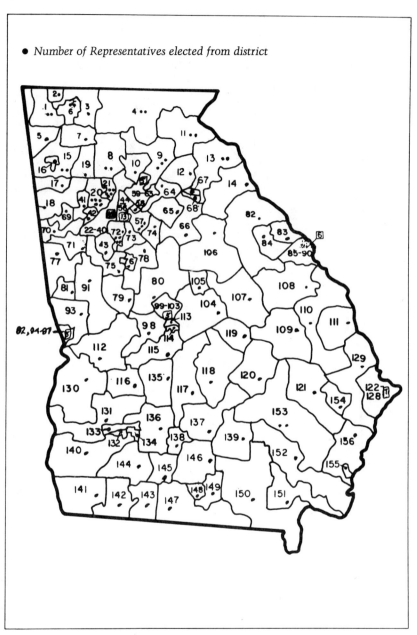

Georgia Representative Map

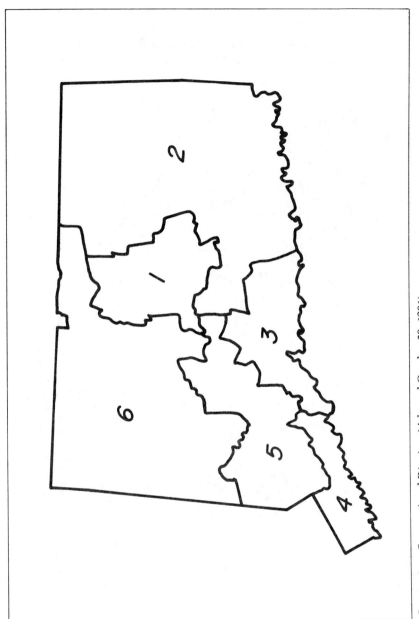

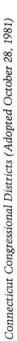

Connecticut Congressional Districts (Adopted October 28, 1981)

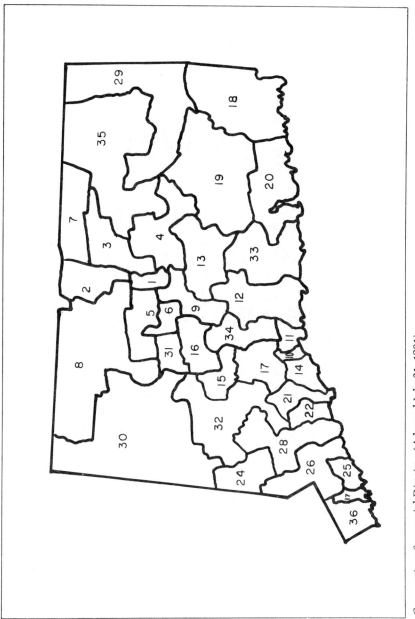

Connecticut Senatorial Districts (Adopted July 31, 1981)

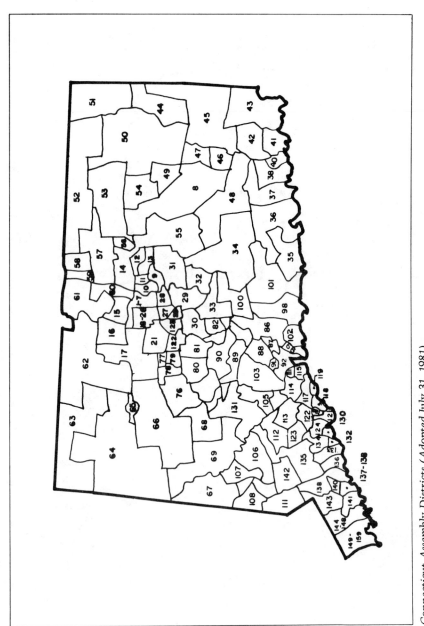

Connecticut Assembly Districts (Adopted July 31, 1981)

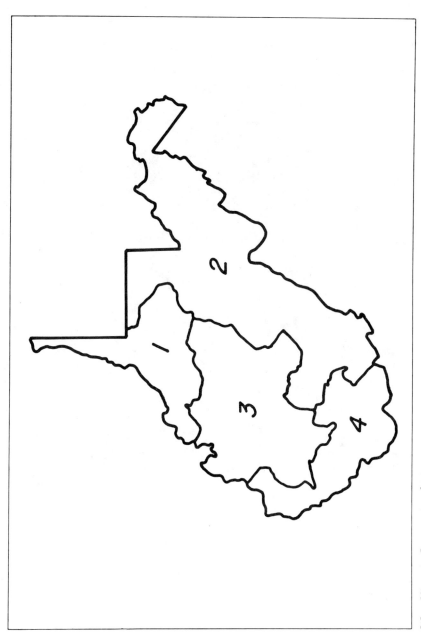

West Virginia Congressional Map

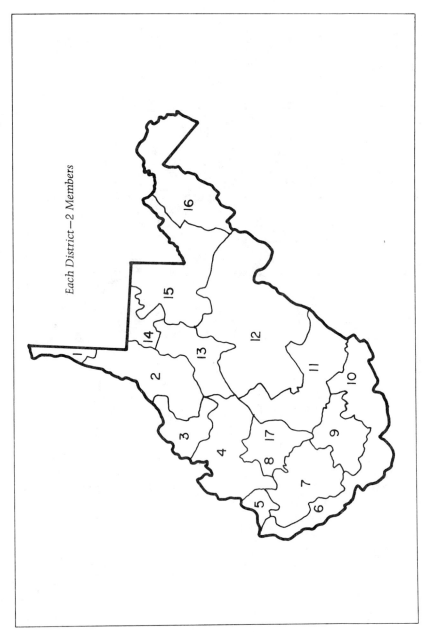

Each District—2 Members

West Virginia Senatorial Map

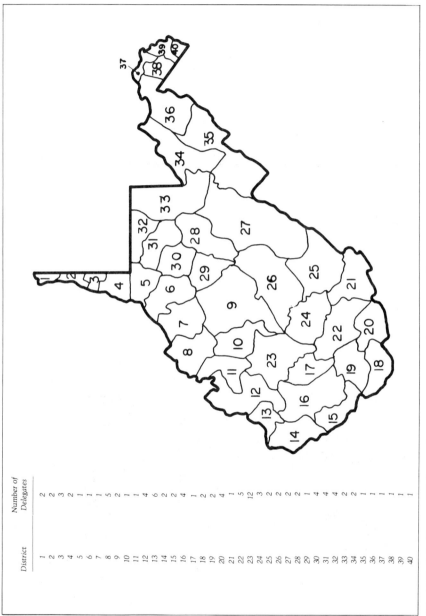

District	Number of Delegates
1	2
2	2
3	3
4	2
5	1
6	1
7	1
8	5
9	2
10	1
11	4
12	6
13	2
14	2
15	2
16	4
17	1
18	2
19	2
20	4
21	1
22	5
23	12
24	3
25	2
26	2
27	2
28	2
29	1
30	4
31	4
32	4
33	2
34	2
35	1
36	1
37	1
38	1
39	1
40	1

West Virginia House of Delegates Reapportionment 1982—100 Members

Chapter 4

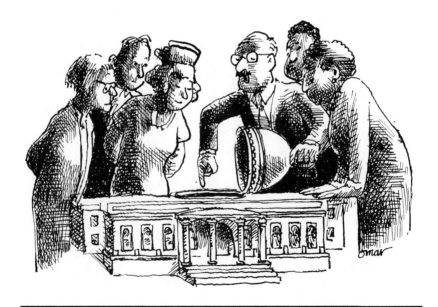

Anatomy of Legislatures

Legislatures, state and federal, are huge fact-finding and educating machines. Because one of the major political themes of the 1980s is the increasing power of state legislatures in the federal process of lawmaking, insight into the mechanisms of this machinery is essential for healthcare professionals if they are to work effectively within the legislative process. Hence, this chapter identifies the components of legislative bodies, both state and federal, the primary positions of leadership, the supporting staffs, and the concepts of seniority and legislative norms. The chapter discusses state legislatures first because most health professionals will not be directly involved at the federal level.

State Legislatures

In addition to the kinds of political districts and the number of legislators elected from them, state legislatures vary from each other in several ways. In some states, as Table 4.1 shows, the legislative body is called a legislative assembly, a general assembly, or a general court. However, the majority of states refer to it as a legislature and to their elected members as representatives and senators. For the ease of discussion, this handbook uses the terms *legislatures* and *legislators*. Some legislatures convene annually, some semiannually. Some sessions are longer, some shorter, and some legislatures have large staffs and nearly full-time members. With the increasing complexity of the matters coming before state legislatures, there is a trend toward increasing professionalism and enhancing the resources and staffing for state legislatures. However, variations remain from state to state.

Table 4.1. *Names of States' Legislative Bodies*

State	Body	State	Body
Alabama	Legislature	Montana	Legislature
Alaska	Legislature	Nebraska	Legislature
Arizona	Legislature	Nevada	Legislature
Arkansas	Legislature	New Hampshire	General Court
California	Legislature	New Jersey	Legislature
Colorado	Legislature	New Mexico	Legislature
Connecticut	General Assembly	New York	Legislature
Delaware	General Assembly	No. Carolina	General Assembly
Florida	Legislature	No. Dakota	Legislative Assembly
Georgia	General Assembly	Ohio	General Assembly
Hawaii	Legislature	Oklahoma	Legislature
Idaho	Legislature	Oregon	Legislative Assembly
Illinois	General Assembly	Pennsylvania	General Assembly
Indiana	General Assembly	Rhode Island	General Assembly
Iowa	General Assembly	So. Carolina	General Assembly
Kansas	Legislature	So. Dakota	Legislature
Kentucky	General Assembly	Tennessee	General Assembly
Louisiana	Legislature	Texas	Legislature
Maine	Legislature	Utah	Legislature
Maryland	General Assembly	Vermont	General Assembly
Massachusetts	General Court	Virginia	General Assembly
Michigan	Legislature	Washington	Legislature
Minnesota	Legislature	West Virginia	Legislature
Mississippi	Legislature	Wisconsin	Legislature
Missouri	General Assembly	Wyoming	Legislature

Types of legislatures

There are two types of legislatures: unicameral and bicameral. Only Nebraska, of the fifty states, has a unicameral legislature. In the unicameral legislature, there is only one house, and all of the legislators serve as one body. Most county and municipal legislative institutions, however, are unicameral. The remaining forty-nine states and the U.S. Congress have bicameral legislatures: two houses, each having separate procedures and leadership. Each house has its own committees and hearings, and joint sessions are infrequent.

Frequency of legislative sessions

Many state constitutions limit the length of legislative sessions, which usually makes the office of legislator a part-time job. At present, forty-two states meet once a year, and eight meet twice a year. Whether they convene once or twice a year, these sessions are known as regular sessions.

In many states the legislature can also meet for special sessions. Special sessions usually occur between regular sessions and handle urgent problems that must have fast resolution, such as the cost-containment issue described in Chapter 2. State constitutions stipulate the manner of calling a special session. The special sessions usually last as long as is necessary to deal with the urgency.

Functions of legislatures

The four major functions of a legislature are lawmaking, representation, administrative oversight, and auxiliary functions.

In essence, *lawmaking*, the first function, is the act of deliberation and resolution of conflict. For example, an obstacle, hindrance, friction, potential improvement, or the like, affecting the public well-being often results in the introduction of a bill to the legislature. The legislators then research and consider means for fairly and legally resolving the issue (Chapter 5 describes this process). Although a majority of the bills introduced each session are not enacted into law, the attention devoted to them enables the legislators to increase their knowledge of the particular subject of each bill and to take positive action in later sessions.

The second function is *representation*. Within the boundaries described in Chapter 3, the people elect the persons who will represent them in their legislative body. Hence, the legislator of a specified district is responsible to the constituents of that district to vote in the best interests of those constituents, to provide information, to be an intermediary for grievances with state agencies, or to be a resource person for constituents seeking employment in state agencies. A diverse constituency will inevitably disagree about the constituents' best interests. The concerns of constituents are generally local and immediate, that is, situations and events that affect them directly at the present time. Since those situations and events affect persons differently, factions arise. From the legislators' point of view, however, the issue is broader. They must consider not just one or two parts but also the entire district and the state. They must consider constitutionality. Your understanding of the broad scope of legislators' responsibilities is essential for effective political action. For example, a healthcare organization that fails to incorporate these broader issues into its communications, lobbying, and negotiating will have difficulty in the political arena. Rather than maintaining a narrow focus on their own concerns, healthcare professionals must condition themselves to consider the larger picture.

The third function is *administrative oversight*. The overseeing of the departments or agencies of the executive branch of the state government is the responsibility of standing, or permanent, committees in the legislature. A major force in oversight is the professional staff for what is often called the Joint Legislative Budget Committee. Through reports from the hearings of standing committees and from the Joint Legislative Budget Committee, the legislators keep informed about the effectiveness and the spending patterns of the state departments or agencies.

The fourth function consists of the *auxiliary functions*. These include electoral, judicial, and constitutional responsibilities. In its electoral responsibilities, the state legislature mandates a system of conducting elections to select major public officials in the state. In its judicial responsibilities, the lower house is responsible for impeachment proceedings involving major state officials; the senate is responsible for the subsequent trial and verdict. In its constitutional responsibilities, the state legislatures have the responsibility for ratifying proposed amendments to the United States Constitution.

Governing by legislatures

Each legislator swears an oath of office. This oath binds the legislators to uphold the Constitution of the United States and the constitution of the individual state. The United States Constitution mandates the sworn loyalty to the Constitution, and most state constitutions have similar provisions.

The state constitution mandates the organization of the state government and delineates the powers of the executive, legislative, and judicial branches. The legislative branch is then responsible for completing the organization. Through statutes the legislative branch creates the agencies in the executive branch. Likewise, it establishes the judicial tribunals — for example, police courts.

The legislature must, after it establishes the structure of government, appropriate funds to maintain the operation of its agencies. The task of appropriation consumes a great deal of the legislators' time and energy. For example, every bill that comes to a vote must have money appropriated if money is necessary to implement the statute.

Leadership

The houses of legislatures across the country are dominated by one political party, either Democrat or Republican. The controlling party then dominates the leadership of the legislature. The important leadership roles within a legislature are presiding officers, party floor leaders, and committee chairpersons.

The presiding officers of the legislature are the president of the senate and speaker of the house. These two officers are the foremost leaders in the legislature. Members of the majority party of each house elect these presiding officers at pre-session organizational meetings, called caucuses.

For example, Arizona has thirty legislative districts. One state senator and two state representatives are elected from each district. Hence, the majority in the senate is sixteen senate seats, and the majority in the house is thirty-one representatives. If the Republican party has the majority of the seats in both houses, then the Republican senators and representatives choose the leaders for their respective houses and make many decisions concerning the leadership of each house.

The presiding officers are able to influence the action in their respective houses in several ways. They have the authority to establish committees, assign members to committees, and appoint committee chairpersons. The presiding officers also refer a bill to a committee after it is introduced. The presiding officers can effectively kill a bill by referring it to more than a usual number of committees. For example, if the bill is assigned to more than four standing committees, it is generally considered dead in that session because it is very difficult to move it through that many committees in one session. The presiding officers also decide when to schedule a bill for a floor vote after it has made its way through the committees. In addition, the presiding officers conduct the daily activities of the floor deliberations; thus, they recognize those who wish to speak and render parliamentary rulings. With all of these powers, presiding officers are indeed influential.

The temporary presiding officers are the speaker pro tempore (or pro tem) of the lower house and president pro tempore (or pro tem) of the upper house. These two positions have much less influence. The speaker pro tempore and president pro tempore are appointed by the presiding officers of their respective houses.

In states having an elected lieutenant governor, the lieutenant governor has the task of presiding over the senate. As president of the senate, the lieutenant governor has the additional power of being a winner of a statewide election, thereby representing powerful elements and groups in the state. For states not having a lieutenant governor, the speaker of the house and the president of the senate are elected by their respective houses.

The floor leaders are generally the second most powerful leaders in the legislature. Party floor leaders in both houses, like the presiding officers, are selected at pre-session caucuses. The majority party elects a majority leader and a majority whip, and the minority party elects a minority leader and a minority whip. The majority leader works closely with the presiding officer and has the responsibility for moving bills on the floor, being a key party spokesperson on majority policy measures, and serving as a party spokesperson for the mass media. The minority leader is the chief spokesperson to the media for the policies of the minority party and leads the minority party in floor debates. In addition, the minority leader presides over the caucus of the minority party.

The majority and minority whips are mainly responsible for keeping track of the members of their respective parties. When a member plans to be absent from the legislature, the member must notify the whip's office. Also, the whips try to ensure that members of their party vote according to the party's stance.

After the presiding officers and floor leaders, chairpersons of standing committees have the third most powerful leadership positions in the legislature. Part of their power derives from their being selected by the presiding officer. The other part comes from their right to decide which bills will be put on the agenda of their committees, to preside over the committee meeting, and to appoint subcommittees.

The number and responsibilities of standing committees vary from state legislature to state legislature. Figure 4.1 delineates those in Wisconsin.

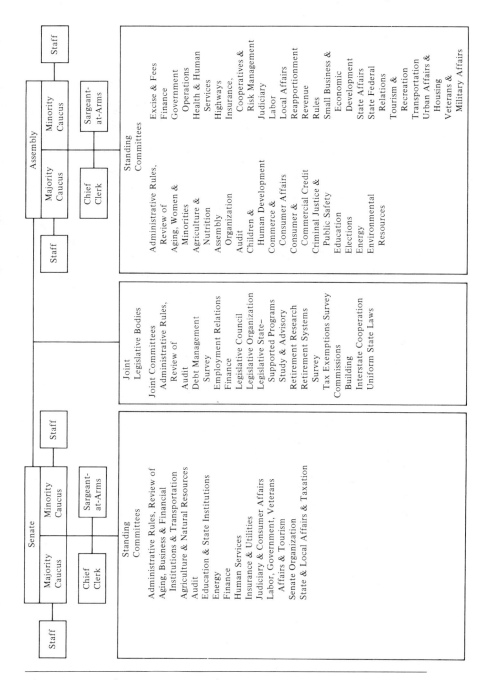

Figure 4.1. *Legislative composition of Wisconsin, 15 June 1981*

Despite differences among them, all standing committees are important because they study bills and make recommendations to the "committee of the whole," which is the entire body of either the senate or house.

The autonomy of standing committees varies in each state legislature, which is the most significant difference among state legislative bodies. A strong chairperson can expand the variety and significance of bills referred to that committee. Furthermore, legislative leaders generally assign bills with jurisdictional problems to a committee that has a strong committee chairperson.

The tasks that the standing committees perform are important and integral components of the organization of the legislature. In essence, the standing committees enable the legislature to process efficiently the many bills introduced each session. Although the establishment of a committee is no guarantee that the legislature will run smoothly and effectively, the effectiveness of a legislature is the result of its standing committees' accomplishing their tasks in an efficient and thorough manner. Because the standing committee can resolve technical questions, it is the best place to perfect the bills. The legislature can then use its floor time to focus on the questions or issues surrounding the bill.

During committee hearings on the bill—which are open to the public, lobbyists, state agency personnel, and other lawmakers—the committee receives and discusses background information about the merits or deficiencies of a bill. The committee eventually votes the bill out of committee or continues to investigate it. Prolonged investigation can kill a bill—it "dies in committee."

Although the standing committees vary from state to state, the houses of all legislatures have a committee that allots, or appropriates, monies and a rules committee. The committee allotting monies, frequently termed *appropriations committee*, is powerful because it decides what monies are available to implement a bill. It can also withhold the money. The rules committee is equally powerful because it is the clearinghouse for bills coming from all the standing committees. All such bills must receive a "do-pass" from the rules committee in order to reach the floor of the particular house.

The party caucus is another part of the legislature and the committee system. In addition to deciding upon leaders and policies of leadership, the majority caucuses in both houses of the legislature act as policy-screening committees for bills. The screening occurs after the bill comes out of a standing committee but before it reaches the floor. The decisions of the majority caucuses will virtually ensure enactment or death for bills moving through the legislative process.

Subcommittees provide another important kind of leadership. These committees may be standing or ad hoc (or temporary). The appropriations committees of most legislatures have a standing subcommittee, but the others are generally ad hoc. Subcommittees do the hard work of taking testimony, making changes in a bill, and developing compromises before the bill goes to the full committee and the floor. In some states, subcommittees are a place for a bill to die. If the subcommittee does not complete its work before the end of the legislative session, the bill dies in subcommittee. Also, a chairman of the standing committee can kill the bill in subcommittee by requesting more and more research and testimony. This maneuver is sometimes called "placing a bill."

Seniority

The rule of seniority exists in all legislatures. The premise that members who return to office several times have more experience and sounder judgment than do new members provides the justification for this rule. Hence, returning legislators receive assignment to preferred committees or retain their assignments from prior sessions.

New legislators serve an apprenticeship, during which they learn the written and unwritten rules of the legislature. During this apprenticeship, they develop some area or areas of specialization through their committee assignments.

A mistake that any healthcare professional might make is to assume that the power of the institution always corresponds to formal titles. In other words, seniority does not guarantee power. In actuality, you need to examine relationships and lines of power. Legislators who do not hold formal positions of power might exert influence through their personal power or expert power. For example, a legislator's calmness and ability to reason an issue without digression often attracts other legislators for a discussion of problems or issues. This influence would be even stronger if the discussion occurs within that legislator's area of expertise.

Legislative norms

Although state legislatures differ in their legislative organization and official rules of procedure, six norms, or traditions, underlie these differences: legislative work, specialization, institutional patriotism, party loyalty, reciprocity, interpersonal courtesy.[1]

Those legislators who do legislative work, that is work at the task of being a legislator rather than seek personal publicity or advancement, gain expanded influence in the legislature. The expectation of specialization requires legislators to develop expertise in a limited number of fields. This specialization gives them credibility among their peers. Institutional patriotism is also important because the public expects legislators to respect the legislature and its processes. Party loyalty is also important because the party caucus needs support for its stance. Although the degree of party discipline varies in each state legislature, assertion of a party opinion from a caucus carries the expectation that all members of that caucus will stay in line. Reciprocity among the legislators carries the expectation that for legislation outside their areas of specialization the legislators will look for guidance from their party members who have specialization in that area. Finally, interpersonal courtesy is important for the effectiveness of the legislature. Interpersonal courtesy creates goodwill among legislators and enables them to disagree without being offensive. Interpersonal courtesy contributes to an environment that can foster objective consideration of broad issues.

The legislative personnel

The staffs of state legislatures reflect the increasing responsibilities of the legislature. Because the workload is enormous, an adequate staff, both professional and general, is necessary if a legislature is to meet its responsibilities and to act as an independent policy- and decision-making body for the state.

Professional staffs do the legwork, research, and paperwork that permit a legislator to function effectively. For example, a joint professional staff, which in many states is the legislative council, drafts a large percentage of the bills, resolutions, and amendments that the legislature considers. Upon request, the legislative council prepares opinions and legal analyses concerning existing law and proposed legislation for the legislature, its committees, and the individual legislators. Meetings of committees and the whole legislature, conferences, constituents, and so forth, leave little time for legislators to attend to the details of administration and research. Hence, the ability to perform rather than party affiliation is the major criterion for appointment to the legislative council.

Another important professional staff is the joint legislative budget committee (JLBC), as this staff is known in many states. The JLBC is the legislators' primary source of budgetary and fiscal information. Its most important function is the analysis of the governor's budget, which includes monies for the regulatory agencies. In addition, the JLBC often has the responsibility for appointing the state's auditor general and a deputy auditor general and for supervising the activities of that office.

The general staff, on the other hand, handles the day-to-day affairs that keep the legislature working. The chief clerk of the house of representatives and the secretary of the senate are the chief administrative officers and are usually the parliamentarians of their respective chambers. Administrative assistants to the president of the senate and the house administration committee, in addition to their various responsibilities, supervise the nonprofessional staff members in the senate and the house, including those in the legislators' offices and the research aides of standing committees.

Both the professional and general staffs are valuable sources of information for constituents as well as legislators. However, many health-care professionals overlook these people. From drafting committees and the JLBC come information about requirements, processes, and the status of specific bills. Librarians are often walking encyclopedias who can save you hours of time. The mail room staff can eliminate a lot of red tape, and research aides can provide insights about particular bills and their prospects, suggest ways to structure testimony, and the like. Administrative officers and administrative aides can provide information about bills, committees, legislators, possible agendas, and the like. These persons are not powerless underlings. Rather, they are very skilled at their work and exert considerable expert and, often, delegated power.

Congress

The Congress of the United States is bicameral, having a Senate and a House of Representatives. The Senate has one hundred members, two from each state. Like the state legislatures it receives its mandate from the U.S. Constitution, and its members swear an oath of loyalty to the United States. Every two years, one-third of the senators face reelection. The membership of the House is 435, a figure set by law. The number of representatives each state has is determined by the population reported in the last U.S. census. The entire membership of the House comes up for reelection every even-numbered year. Congress convenes January 3 of every year.

Legislative functions

Like state legislatures, the first function of Congress is *lawmaking,* whereby senators and representatives deliberate and resolve conflict. The second is *representation,* which differs from that of state legislators in that local representation — the attention to the concerns of constituents back home — must be considered in the light of not only the best interest of the state but also the best interest of the nation. Congress, also, has the function of *administrative oversight.* Like the states, Congress oversees the agencies of the executive branch and funds them. The two major agencies that assist Congress with oversight are the General Accounting Office (GAO) and the Congressional Budget Office (CBO). The *auxiliary* function differs from that of the states in that it includes an *investigative power.* Congress can investigate activities in the executive branch, the private sector, or wherever it believes investigation is necessary. Recent investigations have included the activities of a White House aide, of the Attorney General, and of organized crime. Other auxiliary functions are the rights to approve presidential appointments and to impeach and try federal officers.

Seniority and legislative norms

The traditions of seniority and legislative norms are present in Congress as they are in state legislatures. In recent years, however, some members of Congress have attacked the system. Also, Common Cause, a nongovernmental watchdog organization that works for the best interest of consumers, has been advocating a limit to the number of times a senator or representative can run for reelection. Despite these threats to seniority and despite the increasing numbers of the junior members, the tradition of seniority still operates. As in the states, however, seniority does not guarantee power. Similarly, the legislative tradition of party loyalty has been under stress. Increasingly, members sometimes disagree with their party's stance on specific legislation and vote their own beliefs or those of their constituents. However, like seniority, party loyalty still operates — and in many instances with traditional effectiveness. Along with the rise in independence from party on some issues, interpersonal courtesy and institutional loyalty have slipped at times. Name-calling in chambers and in the press have startled everyone from time to time, as have the misbehavior, violations of the law, and tale-telling of some members. On the whole, however, the majority of the members of Congress adhere to interpersonal courtesy and institutional loyalty. The remaining traditions — legislative work, specialization, and reciprocity — are firmly in place.

Leadership

Leadership in Congress is like that in state legislatures. However, there are several differences. The president of the Senate is the vice-president of the United States. Unlike this office in state legislatures, the function is primarily ceremonial. The president of the Senate has the right to preside and to vote to break a tie. The real leadership in the Senate comes from the majority leader of the Senate, who schedules debates, assigns bills to committees, appoints members of special committees, and coordinates party policy. There are also a majority whip, minority leader, and minority whip whose functions are comparable to those for the state counterparts. The leadership of the House compares to that of the lower house in the states: speaker of the house, majority and minority leaders, and majority and minority whips.

In the Senate, assignment to committees comes from the Democrats' Steering Committee and the Republicans' Committee on Committees. Both parties have a policy committee to determine party stances and strategy. The caucuses for each party are called conferences. The Senate Democratic leader chairs the Steering Committee, Policy Committee, and Democratic Conference. Prominent Republican senators chair the Committee on Committees, Policy Committee, and Republican Conference.

Committee leadership in the House is somewhat different. The

Democratic Steering Committee functions as an executive committee of the caucus. It makes committee assignments, nominates committee chairpeople, and plans party policy. The Republican Committee on Committees makes committee assignments and is composed of a member from each of the states having Republican representatives in the House.

The committee system in Congress is similar to that of the states: standing, conference, select (ad hoc), and joint committees. A major difference in recent years is the proliferation of subcommittees to the standing committees. These subcommittees have increased their staffs and their power, thereby lessening the power of many chairpeople of standing committees. At this time, there are sixteen standing committees in the Senate and twenty-four in the House. See Table 4.2.

The major committees in the House are Rules, Appropriations, and Ways and Means. All legislation except that from Appropriations and Ways and Means must pass through Rules before coming before the whole House (reaching the floor). Rules assigns the terms of debate, for example, excluding amendments (closed rule), specifying wording of amendments, and so on. It can also delay or kill a bill. Appropriations, like its state counterparts, decides whether or not to authorize the money necessary to implement an action proposed in a bill. Ways and Means deals with tax legislation, Social Security, Medicare, unemployment insurance, and import tariffs. The increasing power of the Budget Committee, however, is weakening the power of both Appropriations and Ways and Means.

In the Senate, the major committees are Appropriations, Finance, and Foreign Relations. Appropriations receives appropriation bills from the House, but it can add to or subtract from the funds granted by the House. Finance is comparable to Ways and Means and receives tax legislation from that House Committee. Foreign Relations serves as a watchdog over the president's handling of foreign affairs.

Access to proceedings of congress

While Congress is in session, the *Congressional Record* publishes the proceedings. This resource is usually available in the Government Documents section of university and large city libraries, law libraries, and the law libraries of state capitols.

Congress Watcher is a publication of Ralph Nader's Public Citizen

Table 4.2. *1984 Standing Committee of Congress*

Senate	House
Agriculture, Nutrition, and Forestry	Agriculture
Appropriations	Appropriations
Armed Services	Armed Services
Banking, Housing, and Urban Affairs	Banking, Housing, and Urban Affairs
Budget	Budget
Commerce, Science, Transportation	District of Columbia
Energy and Natural Resources	Education and Labor
Environment and Public Works	Energy and Commerce
Finance	Foreign Affairs
Foreign Relations	Government Operations
Government Affairs	House Administration
Judiciary	Interior and Insular Affairs
Labor and Human Resources	Judiciary
Rules and Administration	Merchant Marine and Fisheries
Small Business	Post Office and Civil Service
Veteran Affairs	Public Works and Transportation
	Rules
	Science and Technology
	Small Business
	Standards of Official Conduct
	Veteran Affairs
	Ways and Means
	Intelligence
	Narcotics Abuse and Control

advocacy organization. It provides current ratings of the voting records of Senators and Representatives.

The Bill Status Office — (202) 225-1772 — provides current information concerning any House or Senate bill. In exchange for the bill number, you can find out date of introduction, sponsors and cosponsors, dates for committee hearings, and where the bill is in the legislative process.

The House Majority Whip's Office — (207) 225-5606 — and the Senate Majority Whip's Office — (202) 224-3004 — can tell you when a bill is scheduled for floor debate.

The Cloakrooms of both House and Senate provide recorded messages concerning floor debate, voting, and scheduling:

House Democratic Cloakroom (202) 225-7400
House Republican Cloakroom (202) 225-7430
Senate Democratic Cloakroom (202) 224-8541
Senate Republican Cloakroom (202) 224-8601

Summary

Although state legislatures vary in size, name, type, frequency and length of legislative sessions, they have similar functions: lawmaking, representation, administrative oversight, and auxiliary. They also are similar in their leadership: presiding officers, majority and minority leaders, and majority and minority whips. Though the names and numbers of committees vary, they all conduct their work via committees and subcommittees of varying importance and autonomy. In their structure, they reflect the structure of Congress. Whether state or national, legislatures adhere, for the most part, to the traditions of seniority and legislative norms: legislative work, specialization, reciprocity, party loyalty, institutional loyalty, and interpersonal courtesy. Within this framework, power ebbs and flows; constitutional and case law provide a foundation for statutory law; and there is oversight for agencies making regulatory law. Political boundaries invite conflict, overlap, and reciprocity. Your awareness of the legislative structure in which these various actions occur will make active participation in the political game more effective than it otherwise would be. With such awareness, you can be on your way to becoming an expert player.

Note

[1]Jewell, M., and Patterson, S. *The legislative process in the United States*, 3rd ed. New York: Random House, 1977, pp. 338–345.

Suggestions for Additional Reading

American Association of University Women, *Community actions tool catalog*. AAUW Sales Office, Washington, DC, 1981.
Balutis, A., and Butler, D. (eds.). *The political purse strings: The role of the legislature in the budgetary process*. New York: Sage Publications, John Wiley & Sons, 1975.

Heaphey, J., and Balutis, A. (eds.). *Legislative staffing: A comparative perspective.* New York: Sage Publications, John Wiley & Sons, 1978.

Jacob. H., and Vines, K. *Politics in the American states: A comparative analysis,* 3rd ed. Boston: Little, Brown and Company, 1976.

Jewell, M. *Representation in state legislatures.* Lexington: University Press of Kentucky, 1982.

Jordan, C. The power of political activity, in Stevens, K. R. (ed.) *Power and influence: A source book for nurses.* New York: John Wiley & Sons, Inc., 1983.

Mason, P. *Manual of legislative procedure for legislative and other governmental bodies.* Sacramento: State of California Legislature, 1979.

Radler, Don. *How Congress Works.* New York: Signet, 1976.

Smothers, F. (ed.) *The Book of the States.* Chicago, Council of State Government, 1977–1978.

The United States government manual, 1981–1982. Washington DC: U.S. Government Printing Office, 1981.

Wasserman, Gary. *The Basics of American Politics.* 3rd ed. Boston: Little, Brown and Company, 1982.

Chapter 5

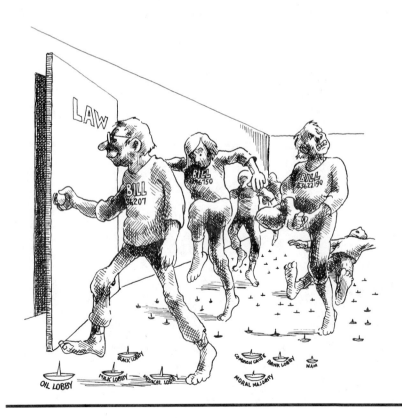

The Legislative Process

When health professionals are actively supporting or opposing proposed legislation, or when they are thinking of proposing legislation, they need to know the legislative process. Too often, however, health professionals think that only a paid lobbyist needs this knowledge. In actuality, the effectiveness of political action increases when all members of a health profession know the entire process of lawmaking in the legislature — from idea to conclusion. Those who know the process participate more in letter-writing campaigns, on various committees of their organizations, in establishing contact with their legislators, and in many other political activities, both long-range and urgent. In other words, people become more involved in something they understand. Although many types of legislation pass through state legislatures and Congress, the type that most frequently affects health professionals is the bill. This chapter, then, describes the legislative process a bill follows, from its possible inception to its possible conclusions, and identifies the other types of legislation affecting health professionals. Figure 5.1 depicts the first part of the process, from idea to passage in one house of a legislature.

Sources

Ideas for bills come from diverse sources. The president of the U.S. or a governor of a state can propose legislation in a letter or a speech. Such executive requests are often highly political because these persons want to further their own goals and objectives and those of their party. Other requests can come from a department within the executive branch or the

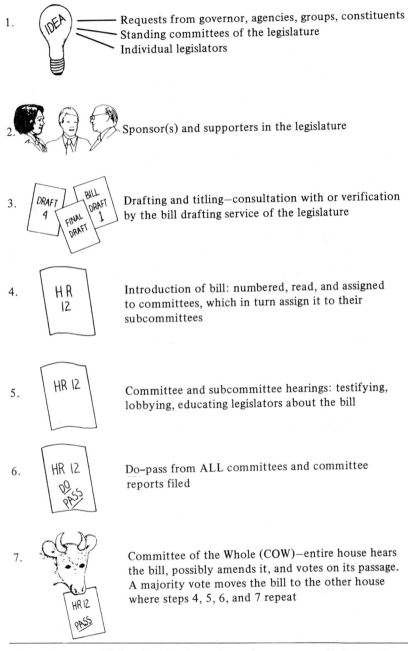

1. Requests from governor, agencies, groups, constituents
   Standing committees of the legislature
   Individual legislators

2. Sponsor(s) and supporters in the legislature

3. Drafting and titling—consultation with or verification by the bill drafting service of the legislature

4. Introduction of bill: numbered, read, and assigned to committees, which in turn assign it to their subcommittees

5. Committee and subcommittee hearings: testifying, lobbying, educating legislators about the bill

6. Do-pass from ALL committees and committee reports filed

7. Committee of the Whole (COW)—entire house hears the bill, possibly amends it, and votes on its passage. A majority vote moves the bill to the other house where steps 4, 5, 6, and 7 repeat

Figure 5.1. *Simplified path of legislation from idea to passage of bill through one house*

legislative council. Such requests usually arise from an apparent need in the area of jurisdiction. This need might be discovered within a department or agency, or it might be something that a health professional or organization has requested or is drafting.

A standing committee of either house of a legislature may also request a bill. Here, again, the committee sees or learns of a need in its area. The request may also reflect partisan interest in furthering goals and objectives of the party whose members constitute a majority on the committee.

The most common source is, of course, the individual legislators. The idea may be a result of a campaign promise, a recognition of the need for new legislation or for amendment or repeal of a statute, or a request from a single constituent or a group.

To decide whether your idea has merit for pursuit in the legislature, you should evaluate certain points. You need to determine that a statute is necessary. There should be evidence that your idea is not already covered under an existing statute. The evidence you gather should be comprehensive and current. The material should be accurate and reliable. Determine whether there is a statute in another state that has proven successful or unsuccessful in meeting the needs that you or your group has identified. Comparison and analysis of existing laws or proposed bills will give you valuable knowledge and provide a model for what to request and what not to request.

Sponsorship

All requests, whether executive, departmental, legislative council, standing committee, individual constituent, or a group, must have a sponsor in the legislature. Generally, executive, departmental, and legislative council requests are automatically forwarded to the appropriate standing committee. For example, requests for legislation concerning health care or a healthcare profession would be forwarded to the committee whose concern was health.

A request from a constituent or group requires more work. For example, if you or your healthcare organization want a new statute or amendment or repeal of a statute, you need to decide where to submit your request. The governor, health department, standing committee for health, or individual legislator(s) are all possibilities, but in making your choice, *be realistic.*

Governors are usually interested in legislation that has wide popular appeal or that furthers their individual or party objectives. They also tend to limit the number of their requests. However, their requests have legislative weight.

Health departments, also, are interested in furthering their own objectives. However, such departments have developed legislative relationships of expertise and commitment. In both cases, governor or department, you need to evaluate how much control you will retain over the content and language of the bill.

Committees on health are another possibility. Here, however, you must convince a majority of the membership to sponsor your bill. This majority might contain both Democrats and Republicans, so your bill should not be partisan.

The usual approach is to seek support from one or more individual legislators. The more sponsors your bill has, the more legislative weight it is likely to carry. First, deciding *which* legislators to contact requires your having some knowledge of the legislators' thinking about health care. You first get to know the individual legislators. Secure any analyses or evaluations that nonpartisan groups might have done. Read any public information that is available. Seek advice from individuals who have worked in or worked with the legislature and who know the members. Finally, have individual members of your group talk personally with as many legislators as possible to get a sense of the way they think on healthcare issues. This information will tell you a lot about a potential sponsor. The fact sheet described for face-to-face contact in Chapter 7 provides a guide for eliciting the information.

Second, after gathering this information, be very careful to stick to objective data. Make as many comparisons as possible, evaluate your information, and label each source: nonpartisan, newspaper, or "one person's opinion."

Because your bill will be requested legislation, your sponsor(s) need to include members of the majority party: as indicated in Chapter 4, a minority member has difficulty in moving any piece of legislation through the legislative process. Ideally, you should have sponsors from both parties. In addition, your sponsor(s) should

1. be committed to your legislation
2. have the time to promote your bill, follow its progress, keep you informed, and provide assistance
3. have the ability to debate effectively on the floor, in committee, or in private (a few first-hand observations at the legislature can verify other people's reports)
4. have leadership ability
5. have expert or personal power

Since only a few legislators will have all of these qualities, select sponsors who have them collectively. Your primary sponsor should have not only commitment and time but also respect from colleagues. Tell your primary sponsor that you will be seeking other sponsors and ask for suggestions. Members of committees to which your bill will go are always wise choices. Be wary, however, of legislators who have in past actions indicated unreliability, self-interest, lack of ability, or lack of integrity. Finally, a legislator whose constituency would oppose such support would obviously not be a good choice, nor would a legislator who has in the past supported groups inimical to your position.

Sometimes, as your bill is taking shape, the governor, health department, legislative council, or an interested standing committee such as the health committee might offer to sponsor your bill. Again, be wary. Weigh the advantages and disadvantages. Such sponsorship might have the advantage of greater legislative force, but it might have the greater disadvantages of increased legislative opposition, self-interest, loss of control over language and content, or loss of a close working relationship. If you have already formed your group of sponsors, switching sponsors in midstream connotes a lack of integrity and can alienate or lessen the commitment of the legislators you have already recruited. When you decline sponsorship, thank the person or group for the support. State that your organization already has commitments for primary sponsorship but that you will tell these sponsors that they can count on the person, department, or committee for support.

Drafting a Bill

Drafting a bill can occur either before or after soliciting sponsorship. Many times, the drafted bill accompanies an executive, departmental, or legislative council request. At the state level, drafting is usually the concern of the primary sponsor of your bill because drafting legislation is highly technical and few health professionals or their state organizations have this expertise.

Whether you wish to draft your own bill or to delineate its desired content to your primary sponsor, you need to get information. Your national organization might have a drafting committee that could provide guidance on language and content. Any successful or unsuccessful models of similar bills in other states can also be helpful. In addition, you need the reactions and suggestions of your organization. Information about the positions of organizations or individuals having power within your state who might support or not support this bill would also be valuable. Such information can guide the phrasing and content. It can also identify ambiguity and areas of disagreement. For example, the word *may* in legislative language denotes permission, the word *should* denotes a recommendation for compliance, but the word *shall* denotes obligation — an action is mandatory. Be certain of your intent before using these words. In any event, remember that your first draft is just that — a *first* draft.

You must also remember that statutes are broad, general rules. Stating things very specifically in your draft will create unnecessary controversy as the bill works its way through the legislative process. The legislative council and legislators will recognize that, should the bill pass into law, legal controversy could result in a declaration of the statute's unconstitutionality because it conflicts with some person's or group's civil rights. Thus, suggestions and reactions, even from your opposition, will help you draft or delineate proposed legislation that means what you intend yet accommodates, as much as possible, other views. It is not uncommon to circulate three or more drafts to your organization, other organizations, and your sponsors before achieving a satisfactory draft.

In this process of drafting or delineating and circulating, you need to consider specific data. Decide what the effective date of the legislation should be. Determine what the impact will be, changing the date if necessary. Determine the cost of implementing the legislation. Estimate the direct expenditures and revenues. In these days of cost containment, analysis of the fiscal impact is essential. Accompanying your final draft or delineation should be an addendum that estimates costs or savings as well as a request for your sponsor to check the estimates for reliability.

Another vital point to consider is the title of the bill. It should be sufficiently descriptive to be useful. It should also stress the positive rather than the negative. For example, consider the options available if you were drafting a bill to protect nurse practitioners from being sued for treating minors for venereal disease. A title such as "Extended Health Services to Children" would be appropriate, but "Venereal Disease Services for Minors" would not. Always clear the title with the bill-drafting service of your legislature.

It is also important to include a few points that you are willing to relinquish. Remember, the legislative process is one of compromise and negotiation. Everyone likes to gain something. Hence, a few extras that you can "reluctantly" relinquish might increase the chances that your nonnegotiable points will remain intact.

On the federal level and in most states, your draft or delineation will go to the bill-drafting service of the legislature. Although it will go under the sponsors' names, it is usually permissible with the sponsors' authorization to maintain close contact with the persons who are responsible for the final draft. In that way, you can ensure that translation into legally acceptable language does not change your intent.

Reading a Bill

Whether you are drafting a bill for a new statute or for repeal or amendment of an existing statute, you must know how to read a bill. Furthermore, the process of circulation requires the members of your organization to know how to read a bill. Such knowledge fosters usable suggestions and reactions.

Identification numbers

Congress. A bill originating in the House of Representatives carries the designation "H.R." plus the number (for example, H.R. 5727). A Senate bill has the designation "S" (S. 1047). A joint resolution has the designation "H.J. Res." (H.J. Res. 2163) for the House of Representatives and "S.J. Res." (S.J. Res. 1503) in the Senate. (A joint resolution is, for all outward purposes, the same as a bill. It is a proposal for legislation introduced in either the House or Senate but has sponsors from both the House and Senate.)

State Legislatures. The designation for bills in state legislatures usually has the initials of the name of the upper or lower house plus "B." and a number. For example, state legislatures that call their upper and lower houses a senate and house of representatives usually designate their bills "S.B." and "H.B." (for example, S.B. 2592; H.B. 3291). If these legislatures permit joint resolutions for statutory legislation, the designation is usually "S.J.R." and "H.J.R." respectively, plus the number.

In all instances, whether federal or state, this designation remains on the proposed legislation as it works its way through the entire legislative process.

Form

Proposed legislation on both the federal and state levels contains five basic items of information: number, date of introduction, the names of the sponsors, establishment clause, and enactment clause.

Congress. A congressional bill displays the information in the following manner:

H.R. 5727
IN THE HOUSE OF REPRESENTATIVES
DATE
PRIMARY SPONSOR (ADDITIONAL SPONSORS)
A BILL

TO ESTABLISH . . .

1.   Be it enacted by the Senate and House of Representatives of
2.   the United States of America in Congress assembled, that . . .

The establishment clause states the purpose of the bill (which is the title), and the enactment clause states the authority by which it will become law.

A joint resolution follows the same format. However, the establishment clause becomes an authorization clause: "Authorizing. . . ." Although the words change, the intent remains the same: a statement of purpose, which is the title. Likewise, the enactment clause of a bill becomes a resolution clause: "Resolved by. . . ." Again, the intent remains the same: to state the authority by which it will become law.

State Legislatures. In addition to the five basic elements, state bills may provide additional information and have a different format. Figure 5.2 illustrates one variation. The parenthetical numbers on the bill correspond to the following items:

1. the number identifying the house of origin
2. the date of introduction
3. the reference title, which names the subject and purpose in shortened form
4. the committee list, which names the standing committees to which the bill has been assigned
5. the sponsors of the bill
6. the establishment clause, here beginning "Relating to . . .," which not only states the purpose but also refers to the statutes being affected by the proposal
7. the enactment clause, which states the authority by which the bill will become law

Line Numbers. Every line of every page of the bill has a number. The series *always* begins with "1," as Figures 5.2 and 5.3 show. Such numbering allows fast reference to specific points and phrases that are under discussion or to changes.

Changes

Additions and deletions comprise changes in a bill. The means of indicating these changes differ. A line through words, phrases, and paragraphs indicate deletion. They are "struck" from the bill or the statute that

STATE OF ARIZONA

35th LEGISLATURE

SECOND REGULAR SESSION

(3) REFERENCE TITLE: board of nursing; sunset
recommendations

HOUSE

(2) Referred on ___February 9, 1982___

HB 2516	**(4)** ⎧ Rules _____ ⎨ GOVERNMENT OPERATIONS ____ ⎩ HEALTH _____
(1) Introduced	
February 9, 1982	

(5) Representatives Kunasek, Thomas, Senator Usdane; Representatives Barr, Cooper, De Long, Hanley, Hays, Holman, Lewis, Messinger, Morales, Vukcevich, Wilcox

AN ACT

(6) RELATING TO PROFESSIONS AND OCCUPATIONS; PROVIDING THAT THE MEMBERSHIP OF THE STATE BOARD OF NURSING INCLUDE TWO MEMBERS WHO ARE LICENSED PRACTICAL NURSES; PRESCRIBING QUALIFICATIONS OF BOARD MEMBERS; PRESCRIBING POWERS AND DUTIES OF THE BOARD; PROVIDING FOR REPEAL OF EXISTING STATUTE PROVIDING FOR A PRACTICAL NURSE COMMITTEE; PROVIDING FOR THE EXAMINATION OF PROFESSIONAL AND PRACTICAL NURSES; PROVIDING THAT THE BOARD MAY SET THE REQUIRED EXAMINATION GRADE; PROVIDING THAT CERTAIN TEMPORARY PERMITS ARE VALID ONLY IF THE HOLDER THEREOF PRACTICES UNDER SUPERVISION; PROVIDING SAVINGS CLAUSE FOR CERTAIN LICENTIATES ON CERTAIN EFFECTIVE DATE; PRESCRIBING GROUNDS FOR DISCIPLINARY ACTION; PROVIDING FOR THE SUNSET TERMINATION OF CERTAIN AGENCIES AND STATUTES RELATING TO CERTAIN AGENCIES; PROVIDING FOR THE APPOINTMENT OF INITIAL PRACTICAL NURSE MEMBERS OF BOARD; AMENDING SECTIONS 32-1602, 32-1603, 32-1606, 32-1633, 32-1635, 32-1638, 32-1640 AND 32-1663, ARIZONA REVISED STATUTES; REPEALING SECTION 32-1607, ARIZONA REVISED STATUTES; AMENDING TITLE 32, CHAPTER 15, ARTICLE 2, ARIZONA REVISED STATUTES, BY ADDING SECTION 32-1646, AND AMENDING SECTIONS 41-2362, 41-2367, 41-2370 AND 41-2375, ARIZONA REVISED STATUTES.

(7) 1   Be it enacted by the legislature of the State of Arizona:
2   Section 1. *Legislative purpose*
3   The Arizona legislature intends by this act:
4   1. To recognize and implement the lessons of the 1982 sunset review
5   of the state board of nursing by the auditor general in order to more
6   effectively protect the public health, safety and welfare.
7   2. That the state board of nursing terminate on July 1, 1992 and
8   that existing Arizona statutes relating to the state board of nursing
9   terminate on January 1, 1993 unless continued pursuant to section 41-2377,
10   Arizona Revised Statutes.

Figure 5.2. *One variation of format for state bills*

1   7. "Physical therapy" means the treatment of a bodily or mental
2 condition by the use of physical, chemical or other properties of heat,
3 cold, light, sound, water, or by massage and active and passive exercise,
4 air, mechanical energy, electrical energy, electromagnetic energy and
5 their necessary physical measures, activities and devices. Physical
6 therapy includes the following:
7   a. Administering and interpreting tests and measurements performed
8 within the scope of the practice of physical therapy as an aid to
9 treatment.
10   b. The administration, evaluation and modification of treatment
11 and instruction.
12   c. The provision of consultative, educational and other advisory
13 services.
14   8. "Unprofessional conduct" includes the following acts:
15   a. Commission of a felony, whether or not involving moral
16 turpitude, or a misdemeanor involving moral turpitude. In either case
17 conviction by a court of competent jurisdiction is conclusive evidence of
18 the commission of a felony.
19   b. Habitual intemperance in the use of alcohol.
20   c. Habitual use of narcotic or hypnotic drugs, or both.
21   d. Gross incompetence, repeated incompetence or incompetence
22 resulting in injury to a patient.
23   e. Having professional connection with or lending one's name to an
24 illegal practitioner of physical therapy or any of the other healing
25 arts.
26   ~~f. Applying or offering to apply physical therapy, exclusive of~~
27 ~~initial nondiagnostic evaluation, screening or consultation, other than~~
28 ~~upon referral of a dentist, podiatrist or physician and surgeon.~~
29   f. FAILING TO REFER A PATIENT WHOSE CONDITION IS BEYOND THE
30 TRAINING OR ABILITY OF THE PHYSICAL THERAPIST TO ANOTHER
31 PROFESSIONAL QUALIFIED TO PROVIDE SUCH SERVICE.
32   g. Practicing or offering to practice physical therapy by a
33 physical therapist assistant other than under the on-site supervision of a
34 physical therapist.
35   h. Immorality or misconduct that tends to discredit the physical
36 therapy profession.
37   i. Refusal, revocation or suspension of license by any other
38 state, territory, district or country, unless it can be shown that such was
39 not occasioned by reasons which relate to the ability safely and skillfully
40 to practice physical therapy or to any act of unprofessional conduct
41 PRESCRIBED IN THIS PARAGRAPH.
42   j. Any conduct or practice contrary to recognized standards of
43 ethics of the physical therapy profession or any conduct or practice which
44 does or might constitute a danger to the health, welfare or safety of the
45 patient or the public, or any conduct, practice or condition which does or
46 might impair the ability safely and skillfully to practice physical
47 therapy.

Figure 5.3. *Means of indicating additions/deletions in a bill*

the bill is amending. Words set in all capital letters indicate additions. In Figure 5.3, lines 26, 27, and 28 are deletions. Lines 29, 30, 31, and 41 are additions.

Legislative Process of a Bill

Since proposed legislation for both the federal and state levels most frequently takes the form of a bill, this section focuses on the process of moving a bill through a legislature. The processes for Congress and state legislatures are similar. Notable differences will be mentioned. For the precise bill-to-law procedure for your state, call your secretary of state's office (see Appendix A) for the telephone number for the legislative information service. This office will send you a description of the procedure.

In most states, as in Congress, a bill may originate in either house, the exceptions being bills that raise revenue and general appropriation bills. One or more legislators may introduce the bill by filing it with the presiding officer of the upper house or the chief clerk of the lower house. In Congress, bills may be introduced any time that the members are sitting. However, state constitutions usually limit the introduction of bills to the first 30 days of a session. In many states a special consent bill permits introduction of a bill after the 30 day limit. Because the number of bills coming before legislatures is increasing, many states now permit filing prior to the opening of the legislative session.

The general process is as follows: a member of Congress introduces a bill, and the presiding officers refer it to one or more committees, which in turn refer it to a subcommittee. The subcommittee holds hearings on the bill, amends it, and sends it back to full committee. The full committee may amend the bill further and then issue a report on it. Once voted out of committee, the bill goes to the next committee to which it has been referred, and the process repeats. The last committee will usually be the rules committee. The bill is now ready for floor action where the legislators debate and possibly amend it. If it passes by a majority vote, it then goes to the other house to repeat the process.

When both houses have passed their versions of a bill, they can negotiate and compromise any differences by modifying the amendments of the other house or by sending the bill to a conference committee. The conference committee tries to arrive at language compatible to both houses. If the conference committee succeeds, and the bill passes both houses, it goes to the president or the governor for approval or veto.

Figure 5.4 shows the typical path of two pieces of similar Congressional legislation as the bills follow the legislative process through the Senate and House. Once a bill is printed, anyone can obtain a copy upon request. For House bills, write House Document Room, U.S. Capitol H226, Washington, DC 20515. For Senate bills, write Senate Document Room, U.S. Capitol 5321, Washington, DC 20510. When requesting a bill, list its number and title. If these are unavailable to you, then give the subject of the bill and the approximate date of its introduction. Congress will send, free, one copy of each requested bill.

To request a bill from your state legislature, call your secretary of state's office (see Appendix A) for the telephone number of the legislative information service. This office will give you the address to which you send your request (usually the mail room) and, if you do not have the number and title of the bill, furnish you with the information necessary to identify the bill for which you want copies. As with Congressional bills, a general idea of topic and approximate range for date will be sufficient for the person to identify it in a computer search. You may also request one from your own senator or representative; you may request one from a sponsor of the bill; or you may request one through the document or mail room. The number of free copies varies from state to state, generally ranging from one to five copies.

Within the legislative process, a bill must pass several critical stages before it becomes statutory law. Frequently, a bill has three readings before the committee of the whole before the final vote. The U.S. House of Representatives, however, has eliminated the introductory reading. This introductory reading consists of reading the number and title of the bill and the sponsor's making a brief statement of its purpose and provisions. The presiding officer then assigns the bill to standing committees. There can be two, three, or more standing committees. Any bill assigned to more than three standing committees is generally dead. Furthermore, in most state legislatures, the chairperson of the standing committee has the privilege of putting the bill on the agenda or of holding it indefinitely.

The standing committee screens the bills and decides whether to move them out of committee. The chairperson places a bill on the agenda

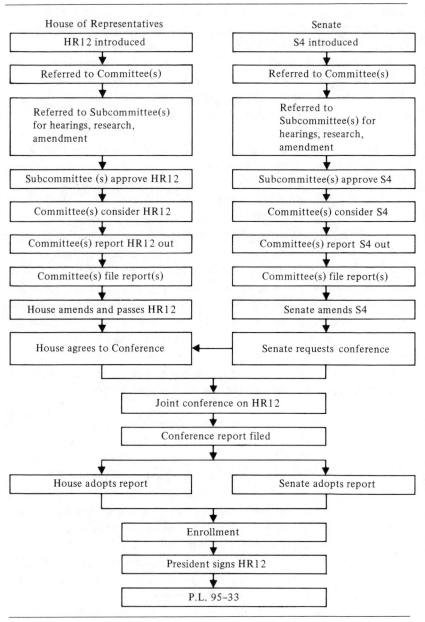

Figure 5.4. *Usual path of legislation from bill to law*

for discussion and possibly a vote, usually with at least a 24 to 48 hour advanced notice that states the time and place of the hearing of the bill. During these hearings the public can speak in support of or in opposition to the bill. Such testimony is described in Chapter 8. Many bills die in a standing committee because the chairperson decides not to place those bills on the agenda.

If a lot of controversy surrounds the bill or if the chairperson knows a need for additional information, the chairperson may assign the bill to a subcommittee. The subcommittee evaluates the bill and holds hearings to gather testimony from constituents. Depending upon the outcome of the subcommittee vote, the bill either returns to the standing committee or dies in subcommittee.

After the standing committee hears a bill, the members will vote to pass or not pass the bill out of committee. Usually, the bill will have several amendments attached to it when it passes out of committee. It then moves to the next standing committee and follows a similar procedure.

In most state legislatures, all bills have to pass through the rules committee, which is classified as a standing committee. The main purpose of this committee is to determine the constitutionality of the bill and ensure the proper form. However, the rules committee also makes policy judgements about the overall aspects of the bill. After the bill passes out of the last standing committee with a do-pass, it is scheduled for the committee of the whole, the entire membership.

There, the bill receives its second reading (first in the U.S. House). The committee of the whole considers the entire text of the bill and all of the amendments that the various standing committees have attached. The presiding officer then allows time for amendments from the floor. At this time, a bill that did not pass out of a standing committee might be attached as an amendment if it is germaine. During this debate and amendment from the floor, the sponsors of the bill run offense and defense for its survival. After the second reading of the bill and its amendments, it is ordered to enrollment (frequently on the state level called engrossment), verification that the bill is identical with the original bill with all adopted amendments.

After engrossment, the bill receives a third reading before the committee of the whole, which then votes on the bill. A simple majority will pass the bill to the next house.

In the next house the bill goes through the same process. Although a bill might successfully pass through one house, it can die in the next one. The bill must pass through the next house without any changes in order to reach the governor or president. But if there are any changes, the bill returns to the originating house. The originating house can accept the bill with the new amendments and send it to the governor or president or reject it and send it to a conference committee.

A conference committee consists of representatives from both houses appointed by the presiding officer. The conference committee negotiates and makes compromises on the various issues in the bill. The members may add or delete material. Sometimes the conference committee cannot agree, and the bill dies. When the conference committee has reached an agreement, it then sends a report to each house for adoption. Each house votes to accept or reject the report.

After final passage of the bill, it is ready for enrollment, the official recognition that both houses have agreed to the bill in identical form. It then goes to the governor or president.

At this point the bill can still be in danger. The bills passed by Congress become law when the president approves the bill and signs it. It can also become law without the president's signature if the president does not return the bill with objections within 10 days. However, if Congress adjourns and prevents the president's returning the bill, it does not become law. This action is called a pocket veto. If the president does not approve the bill, he returns it with objections to the house in which it originated, which in effect vetoes the bill.

The originating house votes on the vetoed bill. If fewer than two-thirds of the legislators vote for the bill, it dies. If, however, two-thirds vote for the bill, it is sent with the president's objections to the other body for a similar procedure. If the bill passes the other legislative body by a two-thirds vote, the bill becomes law. All bills in Congress become law on the date of the president's signature or the passage over the president's veto unless the bill expressly provides a different effective date.

The procedure for governors' signing or vetoing bills is usually outlined in state constitutions. Generally, after the governors sign the bill, it becomes effective 90 days after the adjournment of the legislature unless the bill states an effective date. The bill becomes law without signature if no action occurs during the next 5 to 10 days after adjournment. Governors may also veto bills and return them with their stated reasons for vetoing, and the legislature may override a governor's veto by a two-thirds vote. If the Legislature overrides the veto, the bill becomes law 90 days after adjournment. However, in some states an emergency clause can stipulate that the law becomes effective immediately. Bills containing emergency clauses require the approval of two-thirds of both the senate and house for passage and a governor's signature. However, if the governor vetoes such a bill, then three-fourths of both the senate and the house must vote approval to override the veto.

Summary

Now you have a general picture of the legislative process — how bills originate, what drafting them involves, how to read them, where they go, and what can happen to them. Throughout this process, you as a health professional can have an active part. Whether you are initiating, supporting, or opposing a bill, you can call, write, and visit various legislators who might assist you in meeting your objectives. You can provide legislators with ideas and factual information. You can testify at hearings.

Whichever activity you choose, legislators will appreciate your awareness of the legislative process. Such appreciation can be your first step toward gaining expert power in a legislator's mind: If you care enough to know a process outside your daily experience, you should surely know the facts about your area of expertise.

You, however, might still be reluctant to start. What to say, what to do, and how to do it remain vague. The intent of the remaining chapters is to provide specific help in these areas.

Suggestions for Additional Reading

Arizona House of Representatives. *Arizona Bill.* Phoenix, 1977.
Cowart, M. E. Teaching and legislative process. *Nursing Outlook*, 1977, 25, 777–780.
Drew, E. *Senator.* New York: Simon and Schuster, 1979.
How federal laws are made. Washington DC: West Publishing Company, 1983.
Mason, P. *Manual of legislative and other government bodies.* Sacramento: The Senate of the California Legislature, 1979.

Nathanson, I. Getting a bill through Congress. *American Journal of Nursing*, 1975, 75, 1179–1181.

Powell, S. Legislation scene. *Rehabilitation Nursing*, 1983, 8(1), 37.

Redman, E. *The dance of legislation.* New York: Simon and Schuster, 1978.

Richardson, H. L. *What makes you think we read the bills.* Ottawa, IL: Green Hill Publishers, Inc., 1978.

Shimamote, Y. Governmental influences. In Schoolcraft, V. (ed.) *Nursing in the community.* New York: John Wiley & Sons, 1984.

Wiggins, C. *Arizona legislature.* Phoenix: The Arizona Legislature, 1974.

Zinn, C. *How our laws are made.* Washington DC: Government Printing Office, 1978.

Unit II
Politics in Action

I n Unit I, you learned the rules of the game. You now know the context in which lawmakers work: a description, if you will, of the moccasins they wear. This knowledge is the first step, to change metaphors, toward the increased awareness you need for effective political activity — awareness of the constraints hedging those who make the law — legislators, judges, and agencies. Being aware of the context and constraints, you now know the path: where it starts, where it goes, where the rough spots are likely to be, where a gap in the hedge might provide a way around obstacles. You also know that you will not get lawmakers off the path because the hedges lining it have sharp stickers. So, if you are going to play the game, you too must walk that same path.

Unit II provides guidelines and formats that will enable you to smooth the rough spots, to move the legislators from one side of an issue to the other, to speed them up or slow them down, even to spot a gap in the hedge that might help them around an obstacle. You will learn to negotiate, which is the second step toward increasing your awareness. In learning the process of negotiation and how to apply it, you add to your awareness of context and constraints not only an awareness of the individuals with whom you must work and discuss but also an awareness of yourself. You learn that you are sharing the path and that you need to know about the people who are on the path with you: What are the personal, occupational, and hidden constraints; the motivations; the image? Awareness that such points apply to yourself as well as others will enable you to determine where you can graciously let the other person go first when the path becomes narrow, whether the other will let you go first when you need to, and how you might find room for both of you.

This awareness of others as well as yourself is called, in the field of communication, knowing your audience and your purpose. You determine what you want individuals in your audience to understand and why you want them to. Then you analyze that audience so that you can present the information in a way that encourages reception of the information. Such encouragement often includes granting a concession: You cede a point or two in order to gain a point or two. You are, in essence, negotiating.

Even though you might plan never to be a negotiator for your organization, you need to know how to negotiate in order to communicate with your legislators, to lobby, to testify, or even to participate in a political campaign or run for office. The core of a convincing presentation is the ability to negotiate. Successfully dealing with people requires negotiation. The awareness involved in learning how to negotiate will enable you to use the guidelines and formats of Unit II to their greatest effect. With practice and teamwork, you will find that you can indeed influence the manner in which legislators and constituents walk the path.

Chapter 6

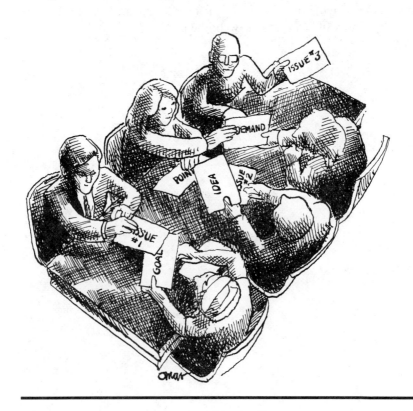

The Art of Negotiating

As Unit I indicated, knowing the rules of the game is essential if health professionals are going to increase their expert power and political clout. But increasing one's clout will create conflict. Rather than thinking that conflict leads inevitably to loss, health professionals should recognize the possibility of resolving the conflict. Positive thinking and creative action can increase the likelihood of resolution. This chapter concerns the resolution of conflict through negotiation. It answers the questions: What is negotiation? When do I use it? Where do I use it? How do I use it?

Definition of Negotiation

In recent years, popular books and magazine articles have boldly headlined that you can get anything you want if you follow six, five, or four easy steps. Since we all would like to get what we want, those books and magazines have sold briskly. But once we explore beyond the covers, we think "Well, yes, that's just common sense" or "I tried that — it doesn't work."

The problem is not the simplicity or workability of the steps. The problem is the classification of negotiation and its contexts. Many of those writings define negotiation as the art of persuasion or communication. In essence, they say that you can win others to your point of view by changing your means of communication. Then they give the idea a context by describing Sue's success once she stopped saying, "I know this will be a problem, but . . ." and simply stated her need: "Would you please pick up the contract (baby, laundry, car, whatever) before 5:00 p.m.?"

However, asking a legislator "Would you please support my bill?" will usually only elicit, "Why?" The legislator will not consciously commend you for your newly found ability to be direct. Instead, the legislator will want facts, cogent reasons, solutions to problems. Negotiating, then, is more than persuasion. It is more than communication. While negotiation does encompass those attributes, there are several others as well.

First, negotiation needs a different definition. Negotiation is *not* persuasion and communication to get what you want. Rather, negotiation is *the effort to resolve disagreements on specific issues. Effort* implies work—expenditure of energy. *Resolve* implies a decision, an end to the matter; *disagreement,* a difference; *issues,* the points of disagreement. In other words, negotiation involves expending energy to decide with finality the differences on various points. That these points are specific implies not only that you can enumerate individual points but also that you decide them one by one. That you *decide* them ends the difference. But the only way you can *end* the difference is to allow the other person to participate. Hence, negotiation is not one-sided, a way to get what *you* want, but two-sided—a way to satisfy both sides.

What to Negotiate

Obviously, any time a difference of opinion exists, you can negotiate. It is not necessary, however, to negotiate everything. In fact, to do so would be a waste of time and energy. To avoid waste, then, you need to know what to negotiate: You research, analyze, organize, and evaluate. Upon completing this process, you are ready to prepare yourself for the act of negotiating.

Research does not merely involve digging out the facts that support your view. Granted, you need those facts, but you first need to know the other person's stance, the reasons for it, and the facts, if any, that support those reasons.

There are several methods for determining a legislator's stance. You can search newspaper archives for press releases issued by the legislator's office and for reports of disagreements on health care matters. The weeks prior to elections are usually fruitful. You can ask questions of those persons who know something about the legislator. You can telephone or visit the legislator, asking the legislator's stance on various healthcare matters. You can create a delegation of three or four persons to formally interview the legislator (see interviewing techniques in Chapter 10). In short, you create as complete a fact sheet as possible (see Chapter 7).

The legislator's stance will probably be apparent, but the reasons may not be. Study the fact sheet to determine possible constraints and influence. The legislator's occupation might yield a clue: If the occupation is one requiring attention to specifications, rules, figures, and fine points, the legislator might be bogged down in the immediate details of the issue and not able to see that the future benefits outweigh those details. Ask of the fact sheet, "Does the legislator's motivation seem to be a need or desire to play safe, to gain acceptance or personal status, or to back the approach that will do the greatest good in the future?"

Then, ask those same questions of yourself and of those holding delegated power in your organization. The answers must be honest. Misleading yourself about motivations, yours or others', can cause some uncomfortable or disastrous moments should the true motives pop up.

After determining a legislator's stance and everyone's motivations, you are ready to research the facts. Bearing motivations in mind, dig for facts that support or weaken your position and those that support or weaken the legislator's position. In your earlier investigation into the legislator's stance, particular facts may have appeared. Research their truth. Analyze their validity. Does the reasoning make sense? Analyze all the facts, looking for relationships and inconsistencies, inferring implications, and the like.

Once you have gathered and analyzed the information, you need to organize it. What seems to be major; what is minor? What is essential; what is not? What negotiating methods might be most effective? Where should you start? What areas have a common denominator?

This categorizing and recategorizing will enable you to determine the various points for negotiation and to evaluate them. Point by point, ask:

1. What are the implications of losing this point? How will it affect us? What will we need to do to accommodate or deflect that effect?
2. Is the point weak? How can I shore it up (if it is your point)? How can I weaken it further (if it is the legislator's point)?

3. What limits surround the point? Do we have enough resources and time? Do we have enough authority?
4. What other groups support which side?

Such questions help to rank the points by pinpointing the ones you can't afford to lose, the ones whose loss won't have irreparable impact, and the ones you are likely, less likely, or not likely to achieve.

Once you have analyzed the points and their degrees of importance and probable achievement, you review and role play. In the review, order the points for best effect and firmly etch them and their facts and inferences in your mind. This review should take several days. Review several times each day. Then role play. Ask yourself questions from the legislator's point of view. Better yet, get someone to play the legislator, deliberately trying to catch you off guard or trip you up. Once you feel comfortable and can maintain your poise and the order of discussion, it is time to negotiate.

Where to Negotiate

Much has been said about the advantage of "home turf": the person in whose home or office the negotiating takes place wins the points. Like most generalizations, this one has its exceptions. The strongest exception is, of course, your preparation. If you have done your homework, determined what is more and what is less important, reviewed and rehearsed, your thorough preparation will bolster your self-assurance. Cling to the thought that you *are* well prepared. We all get stage fright to some extent, but if you recognize it as a normal anxiety for everything to go well, you will find that it is manageable. The legislator will note your self-assurance, and the thoroughness with which you discuss and debate will justify it. The legislator may still not agree, but he or she will be impressed. Hence, thorough preparation can overcome the intimidation you might feel in a legislator's office, the chance of being left without a reply or failing to perceive an error or inconsistency, and the "guest syndrome" — social training that the good guest doesn't disagree or contradict the hostess or host.

The self-assurance that thorough preparation imparts will also enable you to assert yourself and to back up your points with body language. Remember that the guest syndrome has its counterpart, the host or hostess syndrome. If, for example, a chair is offered to you or its placement imparts a feeling of inferiority, say "Do you mind? I would be more comfortable in this chair" (indicating the one you prefer). Or you might say, "Do you mind if I move it a bit? Its position is a bit awkward." With these statements and actions, you have asserted a bit of control over the environment. The host syndrome will usually prevent your legislator from objecting.

Once seated, position yourself comfortably so that your body feels relaxed and can move easily. Obviously, you should avoid lounging. But you should also avoid sitting bolt upright on the edge of your chair, clutching your paraphernalia to your knees. Feeling comfortable will enhance your self-assurance, and looking relaxed will strengthen the legislator's perception of your competence.

Here are several other behaviors that can further enhance your image of competency:

1. Before making your presentation, comment *briefly* on something personal in the legislator's office: a family picture, a trophy, the color scheme, the comfort, or something else. Although this ploy is well-known, it still conveys an interest that can warm the meeting should the legislator choose to respond. If a response is not forthcoming, begin your presentation.
2. If you are a smoker, avoid smoking unless the legislator begins to smoke.
3. Use a clipboard for your papers or a small file folder that opens only at the top—anything that lessens paper shifting and scattering.
4. Keep your voice soft but modulate its pitch. Loud voices and monotonous pitch encourage listeners to tune out.
5. Wear business attire to convey a sense that you are businesslike and competent.
6. Keep your hands still unless you are retrieving or handing papers. Toying with objects, hair, collars, cuffs, and so on, conveys nervousness or childishness.

In short, conduct yourself as if the two of you have equal knowledge, equal respect, comparable skills, and an equal right to be talking in that office. (Remember, your tax dollars help furnish the office and pay the rent.) Such conduct, plus your thorough preparation, will nullify any home-turf advantage.

Your office, offices of your organization, and neutral territory are also possible places for negotiation. Ultimately, however, the best place is the place that best provides for your needs, which can range from secretaries who will retrieve material from files or make copies of documents, to the availability of food, to merely an absence of daily interruptions.

How to Negotiate[1]

The process of negotiating begins with the recognition and acceptance of the constraints of the situation and persons involved. Constraints of the situation are (a) an issue reasonably important to both parties, (b) the need for give and take, (c) a conflict between the fear of losing and the desire for resolution, (d) an uncertainty because the other person's methods are unknown, (e) a real or perceived conflict between both sides. Recognition and acceptance of these constraints will help you to keep your concentration on the issue at hand without losing your objectivity or poise.

In addition to the constraints of situation, both parties to a negotiation desire to maintain a certain image and have certain expectations. First, both of you want to convey the image of a reasonable, fair, and competent person. Your first job is to ignore any threats to your image. Continue to respond patiently and reasonably. Your second job is to maintain the other person's image. Do not question the person's intellectual honesty. Don't leap on the other person's errors with a jubilant "Aha!" Rather, point out the discrepancy saying, "I could be wrong. Why don't we check it out?" or "That source, I believe, may not have the most current figures." Unless there is evidence clearly to the contrary, don't suspect the other person's motives. Accept them at face value. To maintain everyone's expectations of a stable and controlled session, don't spring surprises, deliberately cause problems, or refuse to hear or ask for the other person's ideas. By maintaining these images and expectations, the focus can remain on the equitable resolution of the issues.

Basically, there are two forms of negotiation: trade-off and problem-solving. A frequent ploy is to pad the points with a few that aren't too important in order to have a point or two to trade off. You should not hesitate to do a little padding yourself, but don't get carried away; one or two points are sufficient. Problem solving, however, endeavors to commit the other person to a high-quality solution that the two of you can jointly reach. This approach involves clarifying both sides of the issue, discussing and evaluating possible solutions, agreeing on an optimal solution, and discussing its implementation, which may also be a matter for problem solving.

Major errors in negotiation are failing to consider future impact or needs, ignoring built-in differences between the parties, and over-valuing what you have to trade. More specifically, you need to think not only of your needs as a health professional but also of the future needs of your profession and of health care in general, including those of consumers. You cannot afford to remain unfamiliar with the political process, with the groups that could oppose or support you, or with the constituency that your legislator represents. If you consider future needs broadly and familiarize yourself with necessary elements, then you will be more apt to have a true perspective on the value of your points.

Negotiating a Third-Party Payment Bill

During the Second Session of the 36th Legislature (1984), S.B. 1316, a bill for third-party payment for Arizona nurses, was introduced in the Senate. Prior to its introduction, the nurses had researched the stance and motivations of nursing organizations and their memberships, of the legislators, and of groups that might react unfavorably to the bill. They determined that nurses and their organizations would actively support the bill because they firmly believed it was in the consumers' best interest. Many legislators thought similarly. One group reacting unfavorably consisted of the health insurance companies. Research into this opposition revealed the companies' belief that such payment was unnecessary. The foundation of that belief seemed to be an opinion that such payments would increase operating costs. Research into facts revealed that such payment, authorized in fourteen other states, was safe and cost effective and that it offered consumers a choice. However, discussions of long-range cost effectiveness were to no avail. The companies would not negotiate because they wanted nothing from the nurses.

Despite such opposition, S.B. 1316 passed the Senate handily. In the House, however, it ran into problems from an unsuspected angle. The chiropracters and psychologists, who in 1983 had gained third-party payments until 1985, succeeded in amending S.B. 1316 to include their professions. The representative who had offered the amendment called in IOUs (a form of "log rolling") for support. Thus, S.B. 1316, which had no sunset (a clause stating an expiration date), was burdened with an amendment from those who had a sunset clause. As a result, S.B. 1316 went to conference (see Chapter 5) because the Senate would not accept the amendment.

The ensuing negotiations were hot and heavy. Neither the chiropractors nor the psychologists were willing to budge — they had nothing to lose. Consequently, the representative who had offered the amendment was unwilling to antagonize his constituency. On the Senate side, the sponsors were unwilling to change position on an issue that would probably pass both houses handily in 1985 or 1986. Thus, the nurses had to reassess their position: How much did they want and need third-party payment this year (1984)? Would 1985 or 1986 do just as well? The respective answers, after reviewing their research and polling the nurses, were "very much" and "no."

Having determined that the need and desire for legislation during the current session had not lessened, the nurses then needed to revamp their strategy. They discussed options with their sponsors: What would the sponsors be willing to accept to continue their support? The nurses discussed options with the chiropracters, psychologists, and the sponsor of the amendment. What would they be willing to accept to prevent the nurses from letting the bill die? They discussed with the governor what he would accept. Then, they discussed among themselves what they could live with.

In the end, they sacrificed the absence of a sunset for a sunset in 1989. For the advantage of third-party payment in 1984 when they needed it, they agreed to a sunset in 5 years. They were certain that they would have by that time the figures and other data that would demonstrate not only the nurses' use of the law but also its safety, cost effectiveness, and expanded choices for consumers. They were also certain that a second amendment would not receive support unless the chiropracters and psychologists could present comparable data.

The bill as amended received approval of both the House and Senate; however, the governor, despite previous assurances from his aide, vetoed it on the grounds that the amendment "disregarded" the intent of the legislature's 1983 legislation requiring a 1985 sunset, and his own concerns. The nurses learned several lessons from this experience. In addition to the thoroughness of research into opposition and support, you need to explore who might want to ride your coattails. You also need to explore, as well as you can, what commitments legislators and executives have to other legislators and other groups. The nurses are exploring these questions in preparation for their effort in 1985 to gain passage and signing of the third-party payment bill.

Summary

Negotiation involves knowing yourself, your opponent, your facts and inferences, your issues, and the value and importance of those issues. It involves strategies for creating an impression of equality. It involves awareness of the situational constraints and the desires and expectations of both sides. It involves knowing when to trade and when to engage in problem solving. It is a time-consuming dance in which each side moves slowly toward each other's position through concession, adjustment, and compromise. The theme of negotiation is quid pro quo: one thing in return for another.

Note

[1]We acknowledge our debt to Donald Sparks's book, *The Dynamics of Effective Negotiation*. The categories for the characteristics of the negotiating situation, the five common wants, and the three critical errors gave shape to our personal experiences.

Suggestions for Additional Reading

Cohen, H. *You can negotiate anything*. Secaucus, NJ: Lyle Stuart, Inc., 1980.

Fisher, R., and Ury, W. *Getting to yes*. New York: Penguin Books, 1981.

Ilich, J., and Jones, B. *Successful negotiating skills for women*. Menlo Park, CA: Addison-Wesley Publishing Company, 1981.

Pruitt, D. *Negotiation behavior*. New York: Academic Press, 1981.

Raiffa, H. *The art and science of negotiation*. Cambridge, MA: Harvard University Press, 1982.

Sparks, D. B. *The dynamics of effective negotiation*. Houston, TX: Gulf Publishing Company, 1982.

Warschaw, T. A. *Winning by negotiation*. New York: Berkeley Books, 1981.

Chapter 7

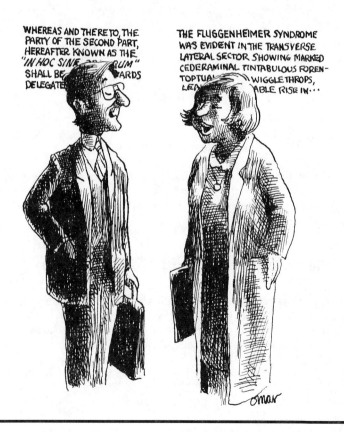

Communicating with Legislators

In addition to its formal structure, the political system has informal aspects. These informal aspects include various kinds of individual and group participation. The common denominator of the various informal aspects is communication. Its purpose is to sway the legislators' views toward or against a specific bill or a general stance. The means of swaying a legislator's opinion include written and oral communication from individual constituents and members of groups, lobbying, testimony before committees, and pressure from community, political, and professional groups. When you as a health professional want to communicate with your particular legislator, members of a specific legislative committee, or other legislators who might be influential in supporting, modifying, or defeating a bill, you have several options: write letters; send mailgrams, night letters, or telegrams; place phone calls; or make face-to-face contact. Whether you wish to communicate as a private citizen or as a member of a group, you need to know the processes and appropriateness of each type of communication. This chapter provides that knowledge and delineates formats that are effective for either individual citizens or members of groups.

Contrary to popular belief, legislators are more likely to be swayed by letters that express individual opinion and provide useful data than by masses of form letters or form wires. The letters that provide useful data and express an individual opinion generally reach a state legislator's desk and have a good chance of reaching a national legislator's desk. The form communications merely reach the designated aide or secretary who counts, measures, or weighs them and reports the number of inches or pounds for or against a specific issue. If the greater amount supports the legislator's view, he or she is of course pleased. If the legislator is opposed to an issue,

25,000 letters giving the same data in favor of the issue are insufficient to change the legislator's mind. Legislators need a considerable amount of data reasonably presented and directed to specific problems or benefits in order to counter the conclusion of legislative research. In brief, although legislators are sensitive to informal district opinion, they want and need data rather than volume.

Consequently, the art of communicating effectively with legislators is crucial to health professionals: effective communication can make the difference between success and failure for your efforts on a particular piece of legislation. An effective communication persuades with facts, reason, and brevity. You must do your homework thoroughly so that you can present the legislator(s) with accurate data directed to specific aspects of a particular piece of legislation in a few written or spoken words. Emotional or vague opinions, threats, or hostile attitudes or tones of voice invite failure, not success.

For all means of communicating with legislators, you need to begin with the following steps:

1. development of a fact sheet
2. decision on the type of communication(s) (telephone, letter, Mailgram, night letter, telegram, or face-to-face contact)
3. implementation of the campaign

Fact Sheet

A fact sheet is a list of data that supports your stand on a particular piece of legislation. The fact sheet should *not* be sent to the legislator(s) because the brevity of the statements can be misleading or cause confusion. A fact sheet is your work sheet, ensuring your thorough understanding of the issue and guiding your communications with the legislator(s). You may need such data as dollar amounts, number of persons in each group affected, number of patients or clients affected, specific detriments of the opposing view, specific benefits of your view, specific weaknesses of your view, evaluation of both the specific benefits that override the weaknesses of your view and the benefits of the opposing view. The fact sheet should contain more data than you will use in a single written communication because you want to have sufficient data for a steady barrage of communications. Also possession of sufficient data will ensure that you will successfully navigate any oral communication, being able to answer the questions the legislator(s) might ask. The following checklist will help you develop your fact sheet.

1. one sentence that clearly states the issue
2. one sentence that clearly states your individual or group position
3. a statement that delineates the status of the proposed legislation (for example, where it is in the legislative process and what appears to be its disposition)
4. a list of the reasons to support or oppose the pending legislation:
   a. financial constraints
   b. groups adversely affected
   c. weaknesses of opposing view
   d. specific benefits that override weaknesses of your view and/ or benefits of the opposing view
5. specific data that support these reasons:
   a. dollar amounts
   b. number of groups affected; names of groups
   c. numbers within those groups
   d. delineation of processes, systems, equipment, or loopholes that have adverse or positive effects
6. a clear, concise statement of the action that you want the legislator to take on the piece of legislation: meet with you or your organization; ask for additional information; convey contents of letter to interested, influential persons; provide you with those persons' names and titles so that you can communicate with them; and so on.

Sample fact sheet

The parenthetical numbers that precede the items on the sample fact sheet correspond to the numbers on the above checklist.

(1) Senator D. has introduced a bill (S.B. 1150) that would eliminate the autonomy of all individual health boards (for example, Physical Therapy, Nursing, and others). The functions of these boards will become the responsibility of an umbrella board.

(2) The state association of each of these professions strongly opposes S.B. 1150.

(3) S.B. 1150 is currently in the Health Committee and will come to a vote in 2 weeks. The committee's agenda designates Thursday, July 16, for this vote. The committee members appear undecided about supporting S.B. 1150. It is likely that the vote will be extremely close.

(4) The bill should be defeated for the following reasons:

    (4) Representation for each healthcare profession would be limited on the umbrella board:

        (5) Currently, each healthcare profession has a state board. Each represents the various areas of the respective boards.

        (5) Fourteen members proposed for umbrella board — means some healthcare professions would not have a member of their professions on the board.

        (5) Each vote only 7.14 percent of total vote.

    (4) Professionalism in jeopardy:

        (5) One representative cannot adequately represent all areas of concentration and preparation. Example: Nursing areas of concentration — medical-surgical, maternal-child, operating room, intensive care, oncology, gerontology, nurse practitioner, education, administration, and so on. Nursing preparation — LPN; 2 year, 3 year, 4 year programs; master's and doctoral degrees. Result — different orientations, knowledge, and skills.

        (5) Existing boards lose autonomy and become advisory committees forwarding recommendations to umbrella board.

        (5) Director of umbrella board makes final decision — can modify, change, or ignore recommendations.

    (4) Umbrella board will cost taxpayers money:

        (5) Operating costs of current state boards paid from licensure fees of healthcare professionals.

        (5) 90–10% financing: 90% for the board, 10% to state's general fund.

        (5) Operating costs of umbrella board will come entirely from general fund.

    (4) S.B. 1150 creates a complex, unneeded layer of bureaucracy:

(5) Existing boards protect consumer:
- set standards
- conduct investigative and disciplinary activities
- test for licensure

(5) Existing boards have effective procedures for resolving conflicts of interest:
- joint meetings
- procedures for negotiation

(5) Umbrella boards inadequate to assume responsibilities:
- fewer members to conduct and oversee activities
- investigatory and disciplinary activities delayed
- potential nonrepresentation, nonvisionary decisions, and conflicts of interest among healthcare professions

(6) Urge legislators to work for defeat of S.B. 1150

Deciding the Means of Communication

Upon completing the fact sheet, you need to decide the type of communication appropriate for the issue. How strongly your group feels about the bill will affect your decision. If your organization developed this piece of legislation, a proactive stance, then the group would utilize all the means of communication in an organized manner. If you or your group opposes a piece of legislation, a reactive stance, you would select your method according to the amount of time available before a vote occurs. A short period of time would necessitate telephone, telegram, and Mailgram. If you have built a rapport with one or more legislators, face-to-face communication would be excellent for quick action. Whatever your decision, you must encourage as many members as possible to participate actively in order to get the best response from the legislators.

Implementation

Letter-writing campaigns

The heart of an effective letter-writing campaign is organization. If you are working as an individual health professional, you should write several short letters, each one elaborating one point from your fact sheet. Allow several days between letters. Mark the writing and mailing days on your calendar. This spacing will not only allow the legislators time to consider fully each point but will also keep them aware of your view and show them your thoughtfulness. If the legislators represent populous districts, as most national and some state legislators do, or if time is short, enlist the aid of several colleagues and personal friends. Your purpose will be to get as much information to the legislators in as short a time as possible. Let your friends and colleagues choose, or assign them a particular point to present. It is most effective to have one lay person and one health professional write on each point so that the legislator will realize that the issue is one of general as well as professional concern.

To mobilize the members of your professional organization(s), you need to send all members a fact sheet along with a cover letter that explains how to use the fact sheet and gives the names and addresses of the legislators to whom you want your fellow members to write. For an individual approach to each legislator, you might attach a separate sheet on which you include pertinent information about the legislator's voting, positions, and activities regarding healthcare issues and those related to health care.

You should mail the information as soon as your fact sheet is ready and follow up with a phone call. If time is short, call the day after the members should have received the information. Otherwise, allow 7 to 10 days before placing the follow-up call. If some members have not yet written, then stress the urgency and answer questions they might have concerning the issue or writing the letter.

Sample Cover Letter. The following cover letter, sent to the members of a healthcare organization, illustrates how to explain the need for action, use the fact sheet, and write the letter.

Dear *(give member's name):*

Senator Doe's bill (S.B. 1150) creating an umbrella board for health professionals will come to a vote in the Health Committee on Thursday, July 16. In order to defeat this bill, we need to get as many letters as possible to our senators and the members of the Health Committee.

S.B. 1150 will not only increase the consumers' cost of health care, which we have been working so hard to lower, but also endanger the representation and professionalism of the individual healthcare boards. I hope you will write to your senator and the members of the Health Committee stating your opposition to S.B. 1150.

To assist you, I have attached a fact sheet and a list of senators, their mailing addresses, the appropriate address and salutation for each, and some of their past positions on health care and related issues. Please keep your letter to one page. To do so, you should select the one or two facts that you can best elaborate or that you consider most important. DO NOT send the fact sheet to the senators. It will be treated as a form letter and discarded. If your letter becomes more than one page, break it into two letters or use legal-size paper.

Please send me a copy of your letter(s) and any responses that you receive so that I can summarize all the letters and responses to keep our members informed of our efforts and the potential for defeat of this bill. Thanks for your help. I will keep you current on the progress of S.B. 1150.

Sincerely,

_____ (Name)
_____ (Title and Organization)

The following list provides forms of envelope address and of salutations appropriate for state and national representatives and senators.

State Representatives or Assembly Members
The Honorable John/Jane Doe
House of Representatives/State Assembly
City, State Zip Code

Dear Mr./Mrs./Ms. Doe:

State Senators
The Honorable John/Jane Doe
Senate Chambers
City, State Zip Code

Dear Senator Doe:

U.S. Representatives
The Honorable John/Jane Doe
House of Representatives
House Office Building
Washington, D.C. 20515

Dear Mr./Mrs./Ms. Doe:

U.S. Senators
The Honorable John/Jane Doe
United States Senate
Senate Office Building
Washington, D.C. 20515

Dear Senator Doe:

Legislative Activity. The following indications of voting, positions, and activities might be the kind of notation that would help the members of your organization to shape their letters to the legislators' political interests.

- Opposed H.B. 2172, which placed physician assistants and nurse practitioners in the same category. Seems to support self-regulation of professional groups.
- Not particularly supportive of healthcare issues per se, but strong consumer advocate.
- Worked actively against the recision of federal appropriations for health care. Concerned about the quality of health care.
- Supported recision of federal appropriations for health care. Works actively to reduce cost of government in domestic areas.

Sample Conversion Sheet. If your membership has not been politically active in the past, you may want to include with the other information a format that suggests how to convert the fact sheet to a letter.

1. Above the salutation, put the bill number (for example, Re: S.B. 1150).
2. Try to tie the facts you select to a legislator's apparent concerns.
3. Use standard English — eliminate as many technical terms as possible. Remember, your legislator probably will not be a health-care professional.
4. Fact sheet items #1 and #2 are appropriate for an opening paragraph.
5. Fact sheet item #3 you need to use with care. Senators A and B are leaning toward opposition to the bill, so you could use #3 either at the beginning or end of your letter to stress the urgency

of their action. Senators X and Y are undecided, so you might want to state only the date of the vote. Senator Z is supportive of the bill (we are opposed), so do not include #3.

6. Fact sheet items #4 and #5 will comprise the body of your letter. Remember to be selective so that you can keep your letter to one page. Other techniques for keeping your letter to one page are legal-size paper, block paragraphs, single space, small margins.

7. Fact sheet item #6 makes an appropriate closing paragraph. We have extended an invitation to Senator A to speak to our organization, so you might want to mention in closing that you hope the Senator will be able to accept the invitation. Your final sentence should offer to supply whatever information the legislator might desire and express your hope that the legislator will support your position. If a legislator requests information that you do not have at hand, let us know immediately so that we can get the information to you.

8. Underneath your signature, type or print your name, address, and telephone number.

An effective tactic for encouraging the members of your organization to write letters is to provide them with paper, pens, and stamped envelopes at a meeting and have them write letters or drafts of letters at that time. Remind them to select one fact to elaborate. Have a few helpers ready to assist the members with details and composition. Although typed letters are preferable, neatly handwritten letters will do if time is short. To encourage individuality of the letters, you could divide the issues among the members. This tactic lessens the chance of omitting an important point and of writing letters that have a form-like quality.

Sample Letter. In the following sample letter, the fact sheet provides the data necessary to stir the interest of a senator whose past political activities have included consumer advocacy. Rather than taking one reason and its supporting data from the fact sheet, the letter abstracts those facts pertinent to the senator's role as a consumer advocate. Hence, the letter does not dwell on the lessening of professionalism per se but rather discusses harmful effects for the consumer: (a) slowdowns in investigative and disciplinary actions and (b) the possibility that persons lacking in expertise in a particular healthcare profession will make decisions for that profession and ultimately the consumer. From the reason "complex, unneeded layer of bureaucracy," the letter abstracts data concerning increased costs to taxpayers and/or consumers.

Furthermore, the letter replaces a technical term (licensure) with standard English because the senator is not a healthcare professional.

The Honorable John Doe
Senator, 2nd District
Senate Chambers
City, State Zip Code

Re: S.B. 1150

Dear Senator Doe:

I strongly oppose passage of S.B. 1150, which will create an umbrella board to assume the governance of the healthcare professions. The state associations of these healthcare professions also strongly oppose S.B. 1150. The existing regulatory boards of each healthcare profession will lose their autonomy and become advisory committees. This action will lessen protection for consumers and raise taxpayers' costs.

Currently, each healthcare profession regulates its members for the public's protection by setting standards, developing and administering tests for licensing, conducting investigations of reported violations, and deciding any disciplinary action. An umbrella board would jeopardize public protection because it will have fewer members to conduct and oversee these functions. Hence, investigative and disciplinary activities will slow down. Some cases may not receive investigation for many months, some even as long as 2 years.

That the director of an umbrella board can alter or ignore the recommendations of an advisory committee can also lessen protection for consumers. This director can regulate a profession he or she may know little about and can miss, for example, the import of a particular recommendation.

Creating an umbrella board and making existing boards into advisory committees increase costs to the taxpayer. Existing boards operate with fees paid for testing and licensing. An advisory committee will retain the majority of the costs — costs of research (whether or not the umbrella board accepts the results), administering tests, and so on. Conversely, the monies to operate the umbrella board come from the state's general fund (taxpayers' money). Raising licensing fees is no solution because at least a portion of the increased cost will pass to healthcare consumers. Eliminating the advisory committees will only require additional staff for the umbrella board and jeopardize the professional expertise that informs recommendations. The solution is to defeat S.B. 1150. It is not needed and will, in fact, lessen protection for consumers of health care and require additional taxpayer dollars.

Although time is short (S.B. 1150 comes to a vote in the Health Committee July 16), I hope you can actively work to defeat S.B. 1150, since in the past you have been an active consumer advocate. I will be happy to supply whatever information you might need to assist you in a campaign to defeat S.B. 1150.

> Sincerely,
> _____ (Name)
> _____ (Address)
> _____ (Telephone)

If a senator's activities and statements have demonstrated an opposition to increasing governments' regulation of business, then the letter could focus on the reason "complex, unneeded layer of bureaucracy" as the fact sheet presents it. The letter could adapt "professionalism in jeopardy" by focusing on the government's jeopardizing the right of those who deliver a particular kind of health care to regulate their profession and to determine what is the best protection for consumers of that care.

Such shaping of your letter to the recipient's interest not only engages that interest but also provides the individuality that carries your letter to the legislator's desk. It is essential, then, that you develop a fact sheet on the legislators who will receive your letter. If your campaign involves only a few people, the fact sheet for letter writing does not need to be extensive. Specific positions on past issues and legislation concerning health care and related topics, and on a few other political interests, would be sufficient. However, if you are helping to mobilize your organization for a letter-writing campaign, then a fact sheet as extensive as the one you would compile for a face-to-face encounter (pp. 124–126) could be invaluable in developing the individual quality of numerous letters.

Finally, legislators can be consciously or unconsciously influenced by grammar, spelling, sentence structure, and so on. A poorly written letter can leave a bad impression of the writer's knowledge of the subject. Letters from individual persons need not be perfect, but the writing should not detract from the content. Letters on the letterhead of an organization should be as perfect as possible, even if they require outside editing, since many traditional organizations that might oppose your position will have professional writers in their employ. The professionalism of your organization's correspondence should equal the professionalism of your opposition's correspondence.

Replies to responses

After you have kicked off your letter-writing campaign, you must evaluate the responses that you and your fellow members receive. Your legislator's reply to your letter will give you an idea of that legislator's stance on your issue and the problems you might have. If a legislator's reply suggests a general sympathy for your cause but states that he or she cannot support you on this particular issue, then this legislator is a prime candidate for a follow-up meeting. This follow-up meeting gives you an opportunity to discuss facts or questions about your issue. If the reply letter includes facts, statistics, and other data that are simply erroneous, you should immediately draft a very polite response giving the correct data and inviting the legislator to call you for additional data.

Sample Response Letter

Dear Senator _____ :

Thank you very much for your response to my letter of July 3 regarding S.B. 1150. I can appreciate your position and would probably accept it as my own if the facts were as you stated them. You noted, for example, that an umbrella board would decrease cost to the consumer of health care. However, an umbrella board operates totally out of the general fund whereas the existing boards operate on a 90–10 basis. The funding for their operation comes only from the healthcare professionals (90 percent of the funds collected), and 10% of the fees go into the general fund. Hence, the operation of an umbrella board will come out of the taxpayers' pockets. The professionals themselves pay for the operation of their individual boards and give the state 10 percent of their fee. This being the case, I hope you can reconsider your tentative support of this bill.

If you need any additional information on this measure, I will be pleased to provide it. Thank you again for your interest and courtesy.

Sincerely,

_____ (Name)
_____ (Address)
_____ (Telephone)

If, however, a legislator persists in opposing your cause even after you have supplied accurate data, you would probably be wasting your time and energy to continue the correspondence.

Telegrams, Mailgrams, and night letters

At times, telegrams, Mailgrams, and night letters are your fastest method of communicating with legislators. There might not be sufficient time for a letter to arrive and work itself through the sorting process before the vote occurs. Or just before the vote occurs, you may wish to remind legislators of important data or state your support or opposition. To communicate with legislators, use the following information. Although the costs will undoubtedly rise, the 1984 figures indicate the comparative expense. In all cases, be certain to use the appropriate envelope address and salutation (pp. 115–116) and to state the bill number (for example, S.B. 1150).

Public Opinion Telegrams. The cost is $4.45 for the first 20 words, except in Oklahoma, and $2.20 for each 20 words thereafter. Western Union delivers the message the same day that you telephone it in. For state legislators, call your local Western Union office. For national legislators, call 1-800-525-5300.

Regular Telegrams. The cost is $8.75 for 15 words and $.39 for each additional word. Omit the salutation. Call your local Western Union office to give the message.

Mailgrams. The cost is $4.45 for the first 50 words and $2.25 for each additional 50 words. A Mailgram is letter size, 8½ by 11 inches. To keep your Mailgram to one page, you would probably want 200 to 300 words for your message. Use salutations. A Mailgram is appropriate for communicating with national legislators when you need something that is faster than a letter yet allows you to give a reasonable amount of data at little cost. Telephone 1-800-525-5300. Upon receipt of the message, Western Union telephones it to a computer at your local or regional post office. The message is transmitted immediately to a computer in the main post office in Washington, DC. It is automatically printed and then put in the regular mail. Allow 1 to 2 days for receipt, depending on the time you telephone your message to Western Union. In some instances, a Mailgram may be as fast as a public opinion telegram. It is generally 1 to 2 days faster than a letter.

Night Letter. The cost is $7.90 for 1 to 15 words and $.26 for each word thereafter. Western Union will deliver it the next morning. A public opinion telegram costs less.

Telephone calls

It is difficult and sometimes impossible to reach a legislator on the telephone. If you are unable to reach the legislator, speak to the legislator's aide. The aide in a state legislator's office might be a secretary. In any case, remember that the designated person has the ear of the legislator and assists in carrying out the legislator's responsibilities (see Chapter 1). It is indeed appropriate for you to give this person the exact information that you would have given to the legislator. Also, the person may give you helpful information about how to present most effectively your position to the legislator. If the person suggests that you send a letter, remember — even if you think otherwise — that the aide knows the procedure and the most effective way to communicate with this particular legislator. In addition, do not expect or demand that the legislator return your call at a certain time or on a certain day. Legislators return calls as soon as their schedules permit.

When calling a legislator about a particular bill, you need to have your fact sheet in front of you along with whatever additional notes that you have made, such as best order of presentation, item(s) to present, and so on. By having this information at hand, you will be able to present your information quickly and concisely and to answer questions with pertinent information. Although you might have little idea of the responses you will actually receive, you can lessen the chance of being caught off guard if you rehearse what you want to say several times and then imagine responses and your possible replies. You should rehearse and create possible scenarios aloud so that you become more comfortable using the words and phrasing, shuffling your fact sheet and notes, and hearing your own voice.

Face-to-face communication

For effective political activity, you should become acquainted with the legislators who represent you. Face-to-face communication gives legislators an opportunity to discuss, ask questions, present their thinking, and increase their understanding of an issue and of your position. Also, many legislators will remember that position better if they have a face to associate with a particular stand and supporting details. The give and take of discussion will help to resolve differences, correct misunderstandings, and provide new data. It will help legislators to integrate your points into their thinking. Two effective forms of face-to-face communication are visits to the legislator's office and speaking engagements for your organization.

Personal Visits. For your first visit to a legislator's office, you might plan to visit all the legislators who represent you. Whether or not you reside in the capital city of your state, visiting more than one legislator would be an effective use of your time and might save you a later trip. If you are going to Washington, DC, you will of course want to visit as many legislators as possible — not only those who represent you but also key members of committees concerned with healthcare legislation.

Such visits will increase the effectiveness of later telephone calls and letters. You will have an acquaintance to write or call, not just a name. By acquainting yourself with your legislators as individuals, you can shape your telephone calls and letters to their particular views, interests, and ways of thinking. For example, if during your visit a legislator seems vague about your profession or some aspect of it, you can immediately provide a few pertinent details and in future calls and letters integrate a pertinent detail or two into the points you want to make. In this way, you can educate without lecturing. Or a legislator might place everything you say in the context of consumers rather than healthcare professionals. Your awareness of this view will help you (in your calls and letters) to relate your points and data to their affect on consumers of health care.

Whether you are visiting one legislator or several, you should know a few procedures that will make your visit an effective one.

1. Do your homework on the legislators. Know the boundaries and nature of their districts. Learn what their previous occupations or professions were and whether they are still active in them. Learn what civic, community, and cultural affairs they have participated in. Know what political parties they are affiliated with and how they voted on recent controversial issues of particular concern to your profession and to healthcare professionals in general. Learn the legislators' areas of special interest in their political careers and what bills they have sponsored alone or with others. For national legislators, you can obtain much of this information from Common Cause or the *Congressional Quarterly*. The offices of newspapers in state legislators' home towns will usually have their political and public resumes. During election years, a call to the local political headquarters of both national and state legislators will provide a plethora of information. For future reference, you might also want to collect such information about the candidates opposing them for political office.

Such detail gives you a context for the legislators' remarks. If you know a legislator is or was a C.P.A., then you will know that remarks about cost effectiveness of health care come not just from a consumer's point of view, and you can shape your reply accordingly. If you know your legislator's political, community, cultural, civic, and other interests and activities, then you can make knowledgeable comments or replies and not be caught unaware should these topics come into the conversation. Furthermore, knowing a legislator's past and present legislative actions and activities allows you to remark thoughtfully on those that have been and are beneficial to your profession.

2. Make an appointment and be on time. If you arrive unannounced, you will probably not be able to make the visit. Legislators and their aides usually have busy, tight schedules during the legislative session. If you are visiting state legislators, the most convenient method of making an appointment is a telephone call. By calling, you can arrange times and

times and dates that are convenient to both of you. If you are visiting more than one legislator, calling will help you coordinate the appointments into a workable schedule. If you are visiting Washington, DC, write a letter to each legislator stating several times and dates that would be acceptable to you. Should the replies establish a conflict, then respond to one legislator explaining that the time and date creates a conflict in your commitments and offering other times and dates.

When you make the appointment, ask the length of time you will have so that you can tailor your remarks to fit the time. It is frustrating to plan a 20-minute visit only to discover that the appointment lasts only 10 minutes. If you are visiting more than one legislator, be certain to allow sufficient time between appointments to organize what you have heard, collect your thoughts for the next appointment, and allow ample time to move unhurriedly from one office to the next. Time between visits should include time for being lost if the visit is the first that you have made to the capitol buildings.

It is imperative that you be prompt for the appointment. Plan to arrive a few minutes early in case the legislator is already available. Lateness will reduce the time available for presenting and discussing your points and will create an unfavorable impression. Since your purpose in visiting is to establish a friendly basis for discussion, an unfavorable impression before you even step in the door defeats your purpose.

3. Accept the possibility that the legislator may be late or unable to keep the appointment. Legislative meetings do not always conclude on time, and informal meetings are often called unexpectedly whenever need arises. If an administrative aide, whether so titled or not, substitutes at your appointment, the visit can still be productive. Present your information as you would have to the legislator. Remember that the aide is knowledgeable and skilled. He or she will accurately report your visit to the legislator and the legislator's views to you. You might even pick up some pointers from the aide concerning modes of written presentation that are most useful to that legislator.

4. Be professional and objective during your visit, whether you are dealing with the legislator or the aide. Dress in a professional manner, maintain a friendly voice and demeanor, and sit comfortably without lounging. Address representatives and assembly members as Mr. or Mrs. or Ms. _____ and senators as Senator _____. Remember that you are probably the

only healthcare professional in the room, so keep the technical terms to a minimum. Explain or define the ones you do use to be certain that you all are working from the same meaning.

As you enter the legislator's office, announce or repeat your name, identify your profession, and the city, county, or district in which you live and work. Offer to be a resource for matters concerning your particular profession and related healthcare issues. Comment on the legislator's political activities that you approve. Avoid attacking or berating the legislator's past or current actions that are not to your liking.

If legislation affecting your profession in particular or health care in general is pending, you may appropriately ask whether or not the legislator has taken a stand. You will then have opened the discussion and be able to make a presentation or comments pertinent to the legislator's response. Whether or not such legislation is pending, determine the legislator's views before you state your own. By doing so, you can shape your discussion to the legislator's thinking. You can present specific information that supports or refutes a particular remark or general view.

Be prepared to discuss one to three issues or points of one issue, depending on the length of the visit. Although the allotted time or depth of discussion might prevent your covering all that you are prepared to cover, you should be prepared in the event that time does permit. A fact sheet will help your preparation. From it, you can select the points you want to cover, decide their order of importance, and have the background, status, and specific data in mind. Legislators *do* like people to suggest solutions. But be certain to *suggest*, not demand. The legislator is usually trying to consider several viewpoints and to select a solution beneficial to the greatest number of constituents. Hence, your discussion and suggestions will be most effective if you include the effects on constituents rather than limit the context to your profession or healthcare professionals in general.

5. A one-page, typed presentation of important points and supporting facts will be helpful. You can refer to it during your visit and leave it with the legislator at the end of your visit. (*Do not* leave your fact sheet. The plethora of data and brevity of statement can cause confusion and misunderstandings.) Be certain to include at the beginning or end of the typed and spoken presentation an offer to supply additional information if the legislator so desires.

Speaking Engagements. Inviting a legislator to a small gathering of healthcare professionals or a formal meeting will foster understanding between the legislator and the members of your organization. When the legislator accepts the engagement, determine whether or not the legislator has taken a stand on the legislation of concern and what that stand is. At the same time, determine the legislator's preferred format. Arrange the program to ensure that members will have a good chance to talk personally before or after the legislator's speech, or both. For example, you could have a 20-minute "Meet the Legislator" session before or after the speech and offer a question-and-answer period immediately following the speech.

Whether the legislator's position on the issue or pending piece of legislation is favorable, undecided, or unfavorable, inviting him or her to speak before your organization can be informative and build rapport. If the legislator's position is favorable, then the members of your organization will have a chance to express their support and perhaps perceive some direction for effectively helping the legislator. If the legislator is undecided, then a speaking engagement becomes an opportunity to provide information that might encourage the legislator to support your position. If the legislator is opposed to the organization's position, a speaking engagement provides an opportunity for the members to identify the reasons for this opposition.

Caution your fellow members not to take a hostile attitude to a legislator's opposition. Urge them instead to adopt an inquiring attitude toward the legislator's position. Each encounter that healthcare professionals have helps the legislator become more familiar with their position. The more courteously and professionally you receive a legislator's views, the greater chance you have of building rapport and of receiving the legislator's support — if not on the current piece of legislation then possibly on future issues.

Appreciation letters

All too often, legislators will work hard and not receive thanks from their constituents or particular persons and organizations that they have helped. Legislators and their staffs (aides, secretaries, and so on) like to feel that their efforts on behalf of others are appreciated. If the legislator has helped you or your group on a particular issue or piece of legislation, it is proper to let the legislator and staff know that you appreciate their efforts, even if a bill did or did not pass, by writing a short note of appreciation. Such notes are also appropriate for thanking a legislator for a speaking engagement.

Your note should be handwritten and not more than three lines in length. The following letter provides an example.

Dear Senator _____ :

I individually and as a member of the Respiratory Therapists Association appreciate your efforts. I'm sure it was primarily your diligent work that finally defeated S.B. 1150.

Sincerely,

_____ (Your Name)

A Successful Legislative Campaign

Increasingly in the last few years, health professionals have initiated legislation. Such a proactive stance indicates the health professionals' awareness of the need to be involved from the beginning in the decision-making process for the benefit not only of their profession but also of healthcare consumers. Physical therapists in Arizona recently took a proactive stance and carried their legislative campaign to an especially successful conclusion. Their campaign illustrates the effectiveness of communicating with legislators.

The physical therapists in Arizona decided that being able to practice physical therapy without referral from a physician would benefit their clients. Hence, they introduced H.B. 2266 in the 36th Session of the Arizona Legislature on February 1, 1983. The legislative committee of the Arizona Physical Therapists Association, Inc., gave top priority to the support and passage of the bill:

Legislative Committee Planning 1983

Support and try to pass Legislative practice without referral.

Review all Bills that may have an impact in Physical Therapy and would favor opposition.

Review Auditor General's report for Physical Therapy Board of Examiners and add input to new changes in the law by the Auditor General.

Report in conjunction with the Board of Examiners.

Require all physical therapists to vote.

Support or oppose any 1984 Legislation from the Auditor General.

Review all Legislation introduced in 1984.

Review all candidates for Legislative Reelection.[1]

The physical therapists next developed a fact sheet concerning the professional education of physical therapists to demonstrate that physical therapists had the education to practice safely without referral:

Physical Therapist Education

The issue of practice without referral is an issue that centers ... [on] a fundamental question. Has a physical therapist received the necessary training to analyze and then attempt to solve a problem? There has been enough of a change in the curricula of physical therapy schools as well as the availability of postgraduate continuing education to answer this with a "yes." Physical Therapists are now taught to problem solve.

This basic education of a Physical Therapist includes eight semester hours of gross human anatomy with total human cadaver dissection, five semester hours of systems physiology, three semester hours of neuroscience — which includes neuro-anatomy with human brain dissection — four semester hours of patho-physiology, and three semester hours of functional anatomy, which includes pathokinesiology. In addition to these basic science courses, the student receives extensive education in the clinical sciences. The professional program is 26 months in length, which includes 6 months of rotating internships in facilities which offer orthopaedic, neurological and long-term care physical therapy. Prior to admittance to the professional program, a student must complete 67 semester hours of prerequisite college work, which includes chemistry, physics, microbiology, college algebra and trigonometry, psychology, humanities, social sciences and the fine arts. The student graduates from a physical therapy education program with approximately 163 hours.

The different types of treatment possible for patient care is rapidly expanding due to advances in all aspects of medicine, and physical therapy education meets this need by emphasizing the recognition of signs and symptoms of medical problems. The physical therapist assesses a problem and then makes a decision whether treatment will be beneficial or not based on this training. It is important to realize that with this knowledge the physical therapist determines which patient can benefit from physical therapy treatments as well as those who should see another medical specialist.

The physical therapists next decided on the types of communication. The types of communication would be telephone calls, letters from physical therapists, letters from clients, professional lobbying, and testimony at committee hearings. Following are two examples of letters from clients.

March 23, 1983

Senator
District
Senate Wing 1700 W. Washington
Phoenix, Arizona 85007

Dear Sir:

I am writing in regard to House Bill #2266, which I support fully.

I have been involved with rehabilitation for a knee injury and feel very fortunate that I have been helped by some very fine therapists in this past year. I would like to be able to continue with this program on my own but find that it is at my physician's discretion. Therefore, I would like to have #2266 pass as I feel it would benefit me, and others like me.

Yours truly,

(Client's signature and address)

Dear Senator,

I'm 14 years old and I have Arthritis in my legs and back, and my family found this out last year. Before I went to Jay Goodfarb, I couldn't walk at all, and I was in the hospital. My aunt, a friend of Jay, and she's also the head administrator at the Maryvale Health Plan, called Jay and arranged for me to have an appointment. And I repeat, my aunt, *not* my doctor.

When I first started physical therapy, I couldn't walk, and now it's three weeks later and I'm able to walk pretty good without a lot of pain.

So what I'm saying is, please support Jay Goodfarb on the House Bill 2266. Because I feel that you should be able to go to a therapist without the recommendation of your doctor. Just so you're able to get help, you shouldn't need the doctor's ok.

And please support him, because lately he's been busy at the Legislature, so he hasn't been able to do as much therapy as I need. So the faster you agree to support H.B. 2266, the faster Jay can get back to work on me.

Thanks for your time,

(Client's signature)

Jay Goodfarb, Chairman of the legislative committee for the association, in his role of volunteer lobbyist, kept in touch with legislators. As the bill progressed through the legislative process, he kept the association and its membership informed of its progress. Consequently, letter writing could be directed to potential problems as they arose, as the following letter illustrates.

April 7, 1983

Dear Senator,

It has come to my attention that Sen. [name] plans to add a floor amendment to H.B. 2266 that would exclude the treatment of back, neck and shoulder problems from the provision of this bill.

I would like to express my strong opposition to this amendment as it is totally inconsistent with the current practice of physical therapy and the training and skill of physical therapists. Physical therapists are trained to evaluate and treat neuro-muscular-skeletal problems regardless of their location in the body. In just my own practice fifty to seventy-five percent of the treatment I provide is to patients with back, neck or shoulder dysfunction.

There are many [treatments of] children, the older population and others that this amendment would severely curtail. [In essence, the amendment would limit] the ability of the physical therapy profession to provide appropriate care to the citizens of Arizona who are requesting this care.

Again, I request that this amendment not be supported. Thank you for your time.

Yours truly,

Blair J. Packard, P.T.
President, Arizona Physical Therapy Association

Throughout the campaign, the association and its members wrote thank-you letters to legislators who gave support to the bill as it passed through the legislative process, as the following letter illustrates:

March 7, 1983

Representative [name]
Chairman, _____ Committee
Thirty-Sixth Legislature of Arizona
House Wing,
1700 West Washington
Phoenix, AZ 85007

Dear Representative _____ :

Thank you very much for your support regarding H.B. 2266. I hope that you will continue to support this Bill when it comes to the House floor.

Sincerely,

Jay M. Goodfarb, R.P.T.
Chairman
Legislative Committee

The communication with legislators came from a variety of sources and testified to the expertise of the physical therapists and the needs of their clients. Without this varied campaign, the years of effort that the physical therapists had spent in building a legislative base, being active in political campaigns by donating both time and money, having an active legislative committee and a volunteer lobbyist, educating the members of their association in the legislative process, hiring a professional lobbyist would not have been sufficient to pass the bill into law for several years.

However, the high level of organization, plus a fact sheet to guide letter writers, a diligent legislative committee and association, and a committed membership resulted in an overwhelmingly effective campaign: the Governor signed H.B. 2266 into law on April 27, 1983. The speed of passage is indeed remarkable — a few days less than 3 months from introduction to signing into law — since the average time ranges from 2 to 5 years. It is a testimony in itself to the preparation of the physical therapists and the Arizona Physical Therapists Association, Inc. As Jay Goodfarb said, "Work, work, work in organizing your strategy. Telephone calls — letters — telephone calls — testifying in committee hearings, and keeping all the mem-

bers of the organization aware of the progress and problems that need immediate action."

Summary

Effective political action for a single person or an organization
requires communication with legislators. Letters, telegrams, Mailgrams,
telephone calls, and face-to-face meetings are all effective means of communication. Ideally, you should visit legislators to establish the legislators'
views and concerns and, if possible, engage them to speak to your organization. The insight that you and members of your organization gain from
such direct meetings will provide a basis for letters, wires, and calls that
focus on a particular legislator's thinking, preferences, goals, activities, and
situation. If you cannot visit, then a letter inviting the legislator to speak to
your organization or a letter concerning a particular piece of legislation can
be effective. If time is short or you simply wish to remind legislators of your
position or the key points of an issue before a vote occurs, telegrams and
Mailgrams are effective.

To communicate effectively with legislators, you need to be thorough and present a professional demeanor. Remember these points:

1. Do your homework. Develop a fact sheet for each piece of legislation or issue and résumés of the legislators' public and political interests, activities, and positions. Shape your communications to the person as much as possible.
2. In all communications, be friendly and reasonable. In meetings,
   dress and act decorously. Give support and approval for legislators' past and current actions that have been beneficial to you,
   your profession, or health care in general. Avoid hostile behavior
   and tones of voice. Berating and challenging legislators' actions
   will create only resistance and make you appear emotional and
   unreasonable. Decorous behavior and apparel imply professionalism and respect for the office that the legislator holds. Your
   dislike of a legislator or of his or her actions is irrelevant to your
   purpose of providing information and specific data pertaining to
   a particular piece of legislation.

3. Present your information clearly, briefly, specifically, and accurately. Keep your vocabulary clear of technical words as much as possible, and avoid a writing style that detracts from the context of a letter.

4. Tie your points to the interests of constituents and consumers of health care as well as to your own interests as a healthcare professional.

5. Write legislators a note of thanks for any efforts that support you and your organization's views—whether or not those efforts are successful. The legislators and their staffs deserve the appreciation, and the note helps to build goodwill.

In essence, then, your purpose in communicating with legislators is to lobby informally for you and your organization's points of view. You must persuade and support by demonstrating your expert power. In this way, you can build personal power and convince legislators to invest their power in your organization and/or the views of health professionals in general. Over time, such efforts will build a traditional power of healthcare professionals.

Note

[1]Correspondence in this section is taken with permission from the files of Jay Goodfarb, Chairman, Legislative Committee, Arizona Physical Therapists Association, Inc.

Suggestions for Additional Reading

Archer, S., and Goehner, P. *Nurses: A political force.* Monterey, CA: Wadsworth, Inc., 1982.

Clapp, C. *The Congressman.* Washington, DC: The Brookings Institute, 1963.

deKieffer, D. *How to lobby Congress.* New York: Dodd, Mead & Co., 1981.

Hein, E.C., and Nicholson, M. J. *Contemporary leadership behavior: Selected readings.* Little, Brown and Company: Boston, 1982.

How federal laws are made. Washington, DC: Want Publishing Co., 1982.

Isaacs, M. Nurse political action: Interview with Marge Colloff. *Advances in Nursing Science,* 1980, 2(3), 89–94.

Jordan, C. The power of political activity. In Stevens, K. R. (ed.) *Power and influence: A source book for nurses*, New York: John Wiley & Sons, Inc., 1983.

Kelly, L. Y. *Dimensions of professional nursing*, 4th ed. New York: MacMillan Publishing Co., Inc., 1981, 383–387.

Molloy, J. *Dress for success*. New York: Warner Books, 1975.

Murphy, T. *Pressures upon Congress*. New York: Barron's Educational Series, Inc., 1973.

Nadar, R., and Ross, D. *Public citizens' action manual*. New York: Bantam Books, 1972.

Chapter 8

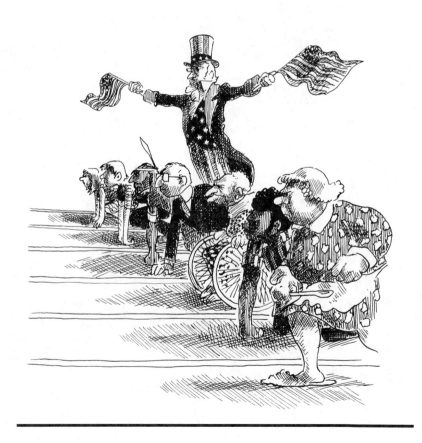

Lobbying

Lobbying is the attempt to influence legislation. Lobbyists try to ease legislation and programs through the legislative process, or they try to block it. To be successful in guiding and monitoring legislation, lobbyists need to know the issue thoroughly. They must be persuasive in their arguments. They need to report the progress of legislation and available options to their organizations. They must be able to negotiate. Lobbying is truly the art of communication. In addition, lobbyists need to gain political expertise and knowledge. They need to become expert in dissecting problems and negotiating to solve problems. Other chapters focus on many of these skills; consequently, this chapter describes methods of lobbying, kinds of lobbyists, and the law affecting lobbying. It provides answers to questions that lobbyists ask themselves as they work through the legislative process and a sample schedule of activities. Finally, it gives pointers for reasoning and for giving testimony.

Methods of Lobbying

In general, the methods of lobbying fall into two classes of communication: the indirect and the direct approaches. The indirect approach involves intermediaries, mass media, constituents, and the like. For example, a friend of a legislator could, in your behalf, urge support of your organization's view. Media campaigns could create advocacy support that reaches the legislator. Many people, including constituents, respond individually. Or a group that consists almost entirely of constituents, commonly known as a grass-roots movement, can inundate its state or U.S. senators and representatives with letters, telephone calls, Mailgrams, public opinion letters, and the like, as Chapter 7 describes. "Nearly every trade association or public interest group of any stature has developed its own grass-roots network to ensure that what its Washington lobbyist says is reinforced by an outpouring from back home. For example in the nursing profession, they have developed the Congressional District Coordinators. For those interests that do not have such a network, a thriving intermediate industry has grown up that promises clients it can take a whisper of public interest and amplify it into a roar of public pressure."[1]

Grass-roots lobbying might also include a mass media campaign — radio, television, newspapers, and magazines — to gain attention for a specific view or encourage a particular action.

Campaign support is another indirect technique. "Campaign contributions to members of Congress serve two important functions for lobbying organizations. Political support not only can induce a Congressman to back the group's legislative interests, but also can help to assure that members friendly to the group's goals remain in office."[2] The processes of these various approaches are included in Chapters 7, 9, 10, and 11.

The direct approach, as the phrase suggests, constitutes direct lobbying — communicating directly with legislators, by telephone or in person, to urge a particular stance or action. This approach has three requirements: access, development of the presentation, and accurate knowledge and expertise. As delineated in Chapter 7, once you have gained access, you can gain knowledge that will help you develop the information that legislators and staffs need for their support of your stance. Your accuracy as a resource person is crucial. Supplying faulty information jeopardizes your political reputation and that of your organization and health profession. It also jeopardizes political success.

The Professional Lobbyist

Professional lobbyists are paid representatives of special interest groups. Their fees differ not only from state to state but also from state to national level. The three major sources for professional lobbyists are public relations firms, law firms, and independent lobbyists. Each of these sources has its advantages and disadvantages.

The public relations firm can generally give your group and its issues high visibility but cannot offer legal services. The law firm lobbyists in most cases can provide you not only with the services you need for your healthcare issues but also with legal services. Independent lobbyists are usually listed in the telephone book under various titles, such as legislative consultants or management relations firms. These independent lobbyists usually have experience as former legislators, or they may have business experience pertinent to a particular area. Independent lobbyists generally have considerable and varied experiences that they can give to the needs of your organization.

In selecting a professional lobbyist, you need to have a clear understanding of your needs. You cannot direct and give effective support if you do not know what you want. Your organization needs to decide the following questions:

1. *What specifically needs doing?* Are there any bills to initiate for new legislation or for repeal or amendment of old legislation? What are they? Are there any bills being introduced that your organization wants to actively support, oppose, or amend?

2. *Do you have a program for the entire session?* For example, you might decide that, in addition to attention to specific bills, you would like to soften the attitudes of some legislators toward healthcare issues. You may decide that specific events or attitudes of the general public indicate a need for closely monitoring legislation throughout the session. You might want to guard against surprises or to ensure that a bill that is dead or dying is not attached by amendment to a bill that is likely to pass (known as *piggybacking* or *paperhanging*). You may want to improve or maintain legislators' opinions of the expert power of your organization and its members.

3. *How much money does your organization want to spend?* The group rather than one person should make that decision because any overspending will require monies from somewhere. If that somewhere happens to be fund-raising activities, you want many members to have a vested interest in the decision. Those persons tend to be more willing to pitch in and help. Also, many members like to know where the money is going *before* it is spent. Generally, a lawyer lobbyist wants an hourly fee plus expenses or a retainer plus expenses. Public relations firms and independent lobbyists are often willing to work on a contingency fee. In some states, however, the

contingency fee is illegal. Evaluate what your organization needs, what kinds of fee arrangements are possible, and what the going rate is.

If you have no program for an entire session, or if your members are not willing to raise money for a full-session lobbyist, consider using a professional lobbyist only for specific pieces of legislation. If your foresee none, consider a volunteer lobbyist.

If your organization decides that it needs a lobbyist and is willing to pay the fee, do some research. Ask other organizations about their lobbyists: What kind have they hired? What are their weaknesses and strengths?

Once you have some names, from referrals and/or the telephone book, interview the lobbyists. You want someone you feel confident about: someone who has the skill, knowledge, time, and interest that match your needs. The advantages of high visibility from a public relations firm or legal advice from a lawyer might be less important than the advantages of personal contacts that an ex-legislator turned lobbyist might have for making last-minute contacts as a bill is coming to a critical stage in the legislative process.

Once you have hired a professional lobbyist, determine what the lobbyist needs immediately and in the future. The lobbyist will probably want immediate background information about your organization, any current or potential bills affecting your organization, and your long-range program, if that will be part of the lobbyist's job. Find out how many persons the lobbyist might need to give testimony at hearings, whether those persons should include clients as well as health professionals, and whether or not the health professionals should include general members as well as officers of your organization. With this information, you can begin your quest for persons willing to testify, provide them with the details they might need to know, and make arrangements for a few rehearsals. You can also, if necessary, prepare to mobilize the membership of your organization for telephone and letter-writing campaigns and attendance at hearings.

Remember, the professional lobbyist cannot do everything for you. The lobbyist can only be a spokesperson for your issues. You and the members of your organization must provide the information and support to enable the lobbyist to present a credible case for your organization. For example, Figure 8.1 displays the letter that the lobbyist for the Arizona

To: Tourism, Professions & Occupations and Health & Aging Committees

From: [Name]

Re: H.B. 2266 — Physical Therapists; Unprofessional Conduct

Date: February 14, 1983

American physical therapy started in 1918. The first physical therapists helped rehabilitate our injured World War I soldiers. In the ensuing 65 years they have effectively treated millions of patients.

The early physical therapists were trained in hospitals for short periods of time. They did not possess the skills to adequately evaluate their patient's conditions and relied on the referral and prescription of physicians before undertaking a patient's care.

As the success and reputation of physical therapy grew, so did its body of knowledge and scope of practice. Today physical therapists are well qualified both by education and clinical training to evaluate a patient's condition, assess physical therapy needs, and safely and effectively treat the patient. Physical therapists are well qualified to recognize when a patient demonstrates conditions, signs, and symptoms that should be evaluated by other health care professionals before therapy is instituted. They also know when to refer patients to other professionals for consultation.

A student graduating from a physical therapy education program has approximately 163 semester hours. Before acceptance in the professional program, a student must complete 67 semester hours of prerequisite college work which includes chemistry, physics, microbiology and psychology. The basic education of a physical therapist includes neuroanatomy with human brain dissection, four semester hours of pathophysiology, and three semester hours of functional anatomy, which includes pathokinesiology. In addition to these basic science courses, the student receives extensive education in the clinical sciences. The professional program is 26 months in length, which includes 6 months of rotating internships in facilities which offer orthopaedic, neurological, and long-term-care physical therapy.

Increasing numbers of patients are requesting physical therapy services. They are frustrated to find they must first be seen by a physician and pay the required physician's fee. This Bill permits practice by physical therapists without initial referral from a physician. California, Maryland, Nebraska, Massachusetts and the United States military services now permit this practice.

This Bill does not in any way reflect an intention of physical therapy to break away from organized medicine. Physical therapists will continue to work for even closer relationships with the medical community. They will continue to see the majority of their patients upon referral from a physician and will, in turn, refer patients for consultation when appropriate. There are many patients, however, whose needs can best be met by the physical therapists alone, and it is felt that the patient deserves the right to choose such care if desired.

Figure 8.1. *Lobbyist's letter to standing committees*

Physical Therapists Association (A.P.T.A.) wrote to the three committees on the physical therapists' bill after its introduction. The first four paragraphs delineate the history of the profession, its growth, and the education and training of its members. The details are many — all of it supplied by A.P.T.A. In addition, the organization supplied the lobbyist with the reason for the bill from the consumer's (constituent's) point of view, an important view to legislators. Finally, in the sixth paragraph, the lobbyist stresses the *absence* of "intent to break away from organized medicine," a question that had, via medicine's lobbyists, been causing a few legislators some concern. Again, A.P.T.A. supplied the content of the response. Thus, with A.P.T.A. supplying information, the lobbyist was able to successfully allay the concerns of several legislators. When you hire a professional lobbyist you are not buying expertise in health care. You are buying time, dedication, and experience in the legislative process.

Volunteer Lobbyists

Volunteer lobbyists, as the phrase indicates, work without pay. Volunteer lobbyists have their own special interests: their professions. Hence, your volunteer lobbyist will be a member of your health profession and, most likely, of your organization. An important point to remember is that *volunteer* is not synonymous with lack of experience. Volunteer lobbyists have influenced many political changes at both the state and federal levels — as long as they had organization and support behind their efforts. To run your own lobby takes time and dedication on the part of the whole organization.

Volunteer lobbyists do the same things that professional lobbyists do. Thus, your volunteer lobbyist should be someone who can frequently arrange to be free of other obligations in order to monitor and lobby during the day. Although volunteer lobbyists usually do not need to be at the legislature every day, they will have telephoning and letter writing to do. And if a bill reaches a critical stage, they *will* be at the legislature frequently, perhaps every day, until the stage has passed. As Jay Goodfarb, the volunteer lobbyist for the Arizona Physical Therapists Association (Chapter 7), said, "Work, work, work, call — write letters. . . ."

Volunteer lobbyists have the advantage of knowing their professions well. Your volunteer lobbyist will have expertise in your healthcare profession. With the fundamental knowledge that the previous chapters supply, your volunteer lobbyist can become adept at the legislature as well.

For your volunteer lobbyist to be effective, you and your organization will need to provide support. Your volunteer lobbyist, like a professional lobbyist, will need to know (1) the proactive and reactive stance of the organization on key issues and bills; and (2) the legislative program for the current session. The volunteer lobbyist, like the professional lobbyist, will need organizational support: research, telephone and letter-writing campaigns, and colleagues to testify at hearings. It is imperative that your volunteer lobbyist receives this support. In addition to increasing effectiveness, it lessens the chances of burnout. Although you can hire another professional lobbyist, finding another volunteer lobbyist is not so easy. And a new one may well be a beginner, who needs to start at the beginning with legislative process, contacts, and general skills in dealing with legislative issues.

To lessen burnout and to facilitate the presence of your volunteer lobbyist not only at critical points but also at the times when a legislator may need information or when there is a need for laying groundwork or monitoring, you might consider a lobbying commitee: one person for the upper house, one for the lower house, and substitutes for these persons. The substitutes would of course need, from time to time, to accompany the primary lobbyist, write letters, and make phone calls in order to ensure a smooth substitution.

Lobbying and the Law

If your healthcare organization plans to use a volunteer lobbyist, or if you plan to be one, you need to know the legal constraints a professional or volunteer lobbyist needs to obey. You can obtain the state laws governing lobbying from your secretary of state's office (see Appendix A).

For lobbying on the federal level, the Federal Regulation of Lobbying Act (1946) and the Federal Election Campaign Act (1971) contain the federal laws that govern professional and volunteer lobbyists. The lobbyist must register as a lobbyist with the Clerk of the U.S. House of Representatives and send the clerk a quarterly report. In essence, the information is a financial disclosure. Upon request, the Clerk will send you the sample forms and current regulations. Section 266 of the Lobbying Act states,

> The provisions of this chapter shall apply to any person . . . who by himself, or through any agent or employee or other persons in any manner whatsoever, directly or indirectly, solicits, collects, or receives money or any other thing of value to be used principally to aid, or the principal purpose of which person is to aid, in the accomplishment of any of the following purposes:
>
> (a) The passage or defeat of any legislation by the Congress of the United States.
> (b) To influence directly or indirectly, the passage or defeat of any legislation by the Congress of the United States.

Section 262 further specifies that the lobbyist will precisely account for

> (1) all contributions of any amount or of any value whatsoever;
> (2) the name and address of every person making any such contribution of $500 or more and the date thereof;
> (3) all expenditures made by or on behalf of such organization or fund;
> (4) the name and address of every person to whom any such expenditure is made and the date thereof.

Also, the lobbyist must not only file, between January 1 and January 10 every year, names and addresses of persons making or receiving specified contributions but also report the total amount (numbers (2) and (5) omitted):

> (1) the name and address of each person who has made a contribution of $500 or more. . .;
> (3) the total sum of the contribution made to or for such person during the calendar year;
> (4) the name and address of each person to whom an expenditure in one or more items of the aggregate amount or value, within the calendar year, of $10 or more has been made by or on behalf of such person, and the amount, date and purpose of such expenditure;
> (6) the total sum of expenditures made by or on behalf of such person during the calendar year.

For every expenditure and contribution, lobbyists must give or receive receipts. They should retain a copy of receipts given for their own files.

Both professional and volunteer lobbyists need to be thoroughly familiar with both federal and state statutes governing lobbying. Noncompliance usually results in large fines, and the lobbyist could possibly go to jail.

The Process of Lobbying[3]

The process of lobbying has four general stages: formulate your program, consider your strategies, implement the action, and evaluate the program.

Formulating legislation

Your goal is to devise an effective program for specified legislative sessions. First, however, you need to identify the issues, defining and classifying specific and potential problems that require legislation and, then, clarifying them:

- What are the pros and cons of each issue?
- Are there any alternative solutions?
- What should our organization's stance be?
- What is the suggested solution?
- Which of these solutions require action from the state board?
- Which require legislation?

Once you have determined the need for and type of legislation, you should identify the legislators who you will need to question. As mentioned in Chapter 7, you should communicate with legislative adversaries as well as advocates and other individuals and organizations who are potential non-supporters as well as supporters. The following questions provide a starting point:

- What do advocates think on the issue?
- What do adversaries think?
- What problems do these legislators foresee?

- What solutions do they suggest?
- What impact do they foresee?

You next need to determine what circumstances, situations, attitudes, and persons or organizations will have an influence on the legislature:

- Who has an interest in each issue?
- What are those interests?
- What is their intent?
- How will they try to influence the resolution of each issue?
- What resources do they have?
- What is their power base?
- Who are their supports and what might their impact be?
- How strongly will they pursue their interests?

Once you have made individual assessments, you need to assess the whole effect:

- How will the circumstances and efforts affect each issue?
- What is the probable final flow?
- What tradeoffs are possible?
- What potential exists for incorporating or combining issues?
- What compromises could reduce conflicts?

Finally, you need to assess the legislature.

- What is the rural–urban split? The party split? The conservative–moderate–liberal split?
- What is the composition of critical committees?
- What political issues are active?
- What slogans or catch-phrases are popular, such as "cost effectiveness"?

Once you have the answers, you are ready to put together a package that has the most potential for passage. To do so, ask:

- Given the current legislature and political climate, which issues should we pursue at this time?

- What similar legislation has previously been proposed in our state? In other states?
- How is our proposal similar and different from the others?
- Under what banner (for instance, cost effectiveness) can we group these issues?
- Do we draft our own bill?
- Who will review the draft?
- What position papers, fiscal or consumer impact statements, or fact sheets are we going to develop?

Once you answer these questions, rewrite the issues as objectives and goals and plan your strategy.

Strategy

Whether you are using volunteer or professional lobbyists, you need to make the following decisions.

- What are our organizational goals and objectives?
- What is our strategic predisposition?
- What human and financial resources do we possess, and which options use them best?
- Is our professional environment competitive or cooperative?
- Do we want to compete, compromise, or cooperate?
- What should our strategic posture be:
    Messenger — inform the uninformed?
    Motivator — activate the sympathetic?
    Missionary — persuade the reluctant?
    A mixture?
- What approach or combination of approaches should we use? If informational, we need to emphasize expertise. If influential, we need constituents with concerns. If organizational, we need a situation to correct.

Once you decide these points, you then decide which legislators to get in touch with. As described in Chapter 7, you must consider the legislators and their staffs, influential persons, other organizations, and public opinion.

Then, create your fact sheets of assessments and background information about each legislator.

Finally, you select your lobbying methods: the ways of communicating with your targeted legislator(s):

- What are the norms of the policy-making body?
- What are the norms of formal and informal legislative procedure?
- What does the fact sheet reveal about the affiliations of legislators and their personal motives and orientations?
- What are our human and financial resources?
- What methods are most compatible with our strategic posture?
- What methods will work best with our chosen channels of communication?

Figure 8.2 provides a matrix that integrates the specific method of communicating (lobbying) with the strategic postures and channels of communication. The strategic choices are informational, influential, and institutional. To dispense information you need expertise. To exert influence you need constituents or consumers of health care who have concerns. To adjust or maintain the parameters of your profession you need consumers of health care who will lack necessary services without such adjustment or maintenance. A specific advocate can be any influential person who has access to legislators. A general advocate can be the media or public opinion as well as an organization. As Figure 8.2 indicates, there are several options. The more critical or controversial the issue, the more methods you should use.

Once the foregoing questions have answers and you have decided on your strategic plan, you are ready to implement the action.

Implementation

In order to implement your plan, you need to stay close to the action. You may have decided by now that your human resources are inadequate and that a professional lobbyist is necessary. However, you should still try to answer the following questions. The answers will enable the lobbyist to incorporate your knowledge with his or hers. In choosing a sponsor for proposed legislation ask:

Method of Lobbying:	Strategy Choices			Direct Channel		Indirect Channel	
	Infor-mational	Influ-ential	Insti-tutional	Legislator	Legislator Staff	Specific Advocate	General Advocacy
Face-to-Face Encounter	◉	◉		◉	◉	◉	
Personal Letters	●	●		◉		◉	
Mailgrams	●			●			
Telegrams	●			●			
Telephone Calls	●	●		●	●	◉	
Testimony	●		◉	◉			◉
Petitions	●			●			◉
Research Reports	◉	●	◉	●	◉	●	◉
Position Papers	◉	●		●	◉	◉	◉
Lobbyist Fact Letter	◉	◉	●	●	◉	●	●
Letters to the Editor		●		●			●
News Releases		◉	◉	●			◉
Talk Shows		●					●
Speeches		◉					◉
Public Demonstrations		●		●			◉
Litigation			◉	●			●

◉ Top Methods

Figure 8.2. *Method strategy/channel matrix[3] for lobbyists*

- Which leading legislators are most likely to support our cause?
- Which one is best for our bill?
- Which one is most influential?
- Which one is closest to critical committees?
- Which one has the time and energy to devote to passage?
- What will be the political cost of this support?

For broadening your support, ask:

- What two or more members should we approach on the pivotal legislative committee (see Chapter 5)?
- What bicameral support can we get?
- What bipartisan, executive, or other support can we encourage?

In monitoring the bill, you need to decide

- How often should regular communication with legislator(s) occur?
- What specific events should signal special efforts in communication?
- How formal, informal, personal, impersonal should each communication be?

and ask:

- What issues are acceptable?
- What is being debated?
- What legislative camps have formed?
- How can we help our legislative supporters?
- How can we influence the uncommitted?

In dealing with adversaries, ask:

- What is their formal position?
- How can it best be debated?
- What is the real issue?
- How can we best disclose this issue or disarm it?
- What are their tactics and how should we counter them?

• How can their legislative support best be eroded, countered, restrained, or neutralized?

However, don't become so involved with the details that you forget the generalities. Keep track of the bill's actual progress:

• Where is the bill in the legislative process?
• What problems do you anticipate at the next level?
• What amendments have been or might be proposed, and what support do they have among the legislators?

As you try to broaden the base of support for a bill and monitor its progress, negotiation and compromise are frequently necessary. As described in Chapter 6, negotiation involves keeping your losses to a minimum and protecting your major issues. Answers to the following questions can help you or your professional lobbyist negotiate successfully:

1. What amendment can we propose to counter that proposed amendment, which would have a major impact on the bill?
2. What legislators of the committee can we lobby for support of our amendment?
3. When should our amendment be introduced?
4. What compromises can we negotiate with our adversaries and draft as amendments?

Evaluation

As you broaden the base of support, monitor the progress of the bill, and negotiate during the process of shepherding a bill through the legislative process, you need to evaluate the process. At the end of the legislative session, you need to evaluate the legislative process and the legislative program.

The following questions will help you evaluate the legislative process:

1. Were the strategies and methods appropriate to accomplish our goal?

2. Did we follow our plan of action?
3. Did we negotiate effectively?
4. What were our strengths?
5. What were our weaknesses?

To evaluate the legislative program, ask:

1. What impact will the legislation passed this session have on the consumer of healthcare services?
2. What impact will the legislation passed this session have on our profession?
3. What issues need to be incorporated into the next session?

In general, there are fifteen activities in the process of lobbying. You can loosely schedule these activities for action during presession, session, and postsession. Figure 8.3 displays this scheduling. As a new lobbyist,

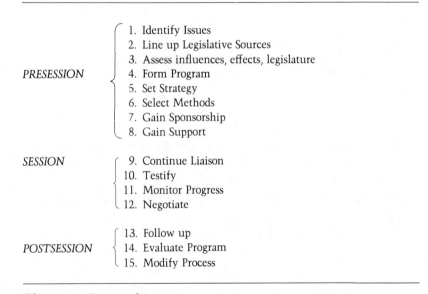

PRESESSION
   1. Identify Issues
   2. Line up Legislative Sources
   3. Assess influences, effects, legislature
   4. Form Program
   5. Set Strategy
   6. Select Methods
   7. Gain Sponsorship
   8. Gain Support

SESSION
   9. Continue Liaison
  10. Testify
  11. Monitor Progress
  12. Negotiate

POSTSESSION
  13. Follow up
  14. Evaluate Program
  15. Modify Process

Figure 8.3. *Timing of activities*

you might achieve item 7, gaining sponsorship, at the very beginning of a session. Item 8, gaining support, you might achieve toward the beginning and as your bill progresses. As you gain experience with the process and acquaintance with legislators, you will try to gain sponsors and support prior to the session.

Argument

Part of your success in lobbying will derive from your ability to argue your position. Such arguments usually fall into four categories:

1. how the health professionals' position will enhance people's lives
2. how the health professionals' position will save money or stimulate business
3. why the health professionals' position is morally right
4. how the facts justify the health professionals' position

Health professionals should be concerned not only with their own arguments but the arguments of opponents as well. Sometimes it is strategically important not to continue to press your points but to attack your opponent's arguments. The following list of logical fallacies will help pinpoint problems of truth and validity in an opponent's or your own argument:

1. Faulty premises: beginning the argument with an unwarranted assumption.
   a. Unqualified, or sweeping, generalization, generally a result of oversimplification. Argument excludes relevant considerations, thereby making the point at issue appear to be more easily settled than is actually the case. *Vitamins are good for you. Milk contains vitamins. Therefore, you should drink milk. (And if you are allergic?)*
   b. False assumption — beginning an argument with an erroneous premise. *Beginning a discussion of nutrition with the assumption that carbohydrates are not really necessary.*

 c. Contradictory premises — if they contradict, you have no argument. *I contend that the bill is terrible; however, without its provisions the consumer would suffer.*
2. Circular argument — one assumes the truth of something that one is setting out to prove. The arguer-in-a-circle offers as proof of his first proposition a second proposition which he can prove only by proving the first proposition. *People who are sick don't take care of themselves because if they took care of themselves they wouldn't be sick.*
3. Begging the question — assumes that which needs to be proved. *Vitamin C is helpful because it reduces the incidence of cancer. (Researchers have yet to prove that Vitamin C reduces the incidence.)*
4. Post hoc (post hoc, ergo propter hoc) — after this, therefore because of this. Because event B follows event A, one assumes event B results from A. *I went to the hospital following the installation of a heliport at the hospital. That is why my bill is so high.*
5. False placement of cause — a slight variation of post hoc. Because A preceeds B, A causes B. *I don't wash my car on weekends because every time I do, it rains.*
6. Either-or — a choice between two extremes, when in reality more than two possibilities exist. The alternatives between the extremes are ignored. *Joe doesn't fly his American flag on the Fourth of July. Joe is a traitor to the United States. (In actuality it is entirely possible Joe loves and respects the United States.) If we elect Jones president, we will go to war. We won't elect Jones. Therefore, we won't go to war.*
7. Appealing unfairly to prejudices and sympathies — playing upon hopes, fears, likes, dislikes, sense of pity: in short, emotions. This is closely related to the either-or fallacy.
 a. *Voice of doom — If you vote for the XXX party, you're voting for economic collapse.*
 b. *Bleeding heart — Unless you contribute to our charity, thousands of little children will starve.*
8. Hasty generalization — using too few instances to support a conclusion.
On the first day of school, you see a nursing student rudely

bump into a classmate in the corridor. A week later you see two other nursing students elbow their way to the front of a cafeteria line. Immediately you generalize: "Nursing Students! None of them have any manners." The error here consists of treating nursing students as if they were objects made to exact specifications. You might be justified in selecting three pencils at random from a lot made to specification and generalizing on the quality of the lot, but you cannot generalize from the behavior of three nursing students. You would have to study a great many more students, and even then you would have to qualify the generalization in some way.

9. False analogy — because one thing (A) has certain attributes in common with another thing (B) one assumes that A will resemble B in some other attribute.

   If you drop a raw egg in alcohol, the alcohol ruins the egg. In the same way, if you drink alcoholic beverages, the tissues of your stomach will be destroyed.

   A false analogy may err in making comparisons that are only superficial. It may also dwell upon the similarities, ignoring the differences. Or it may continue the analogy beyond the point at which it breaks down.

10. *Equivocation* — using the same term, but shifting the meaning. *Using disinterested to mean, first, "objective." Then later in the discussion, shifting the meaning, without notifying your audience, to "uninterested."*

    Disinterested people are objective. (able to refrain from making biased judgements) John is disinterested. (able to avoid bias) Therefore, John is not interested. (without interest)

11. *Discrediting the opposition* (argument ad hominem) — telling the audience not to listen to the other side of the question because its proponents are stupid, dishonest, and subversive. All of these charges are irrelevant. They usually appeal to the audience's prejudices. The other side of the question may or may not stand on its own merits, the only true basis for judgement.

12. *Stacking the cards* — distorting or falsifying the evidence to strengthen one's position. Such tampering is usually deliberate, but an author/speaker with a strong personal bias might do it unconsciously.

a. misstating facts
b. misquoting an authority (altering the words or taking them out of context)
c. misinterpreting facts or quotations
d. omitting relevant evidence (perhaps the most common form of card stacking: a person presents those facts which fit the thesis, ignoring those which conflict with it).
13. *Using irrelevant materials* — presenting materials that have no connection with the original subject. This fallacy might seem too obvious a violation of logic to escape detection, but it occurs frequently in argument and persuasion, especially if the person has strong feelings about the subject.
a. irrelevant thesis — shifting the grounds of an argument from the original topic to one that is unrelated but more easily defended, for example, setting out to prove that smoking is sinful but gradually shifting to the thesis that smoking may be injurious to one's health.
b. irrelevant evidence — introducing materials having no bearing on the topic but which may sway the audience's opinion, for example, supposedly discussing the inadequacies of a bill but dwelling at length on the amount of time and effort put into it and the incompetence of the drafter.
c. irrelevant conclusion — arriving at a final decision that contradicts the facts, for example, piling up evidence that a two-party system is desirable in the South, but then announcing that a one-party system is nevertheless preferable or arriving at a conclusion that is a non sequitur.
   Stating that present public officials are corrupt and then deciding that we shall, therefore, have a change of administration after the next election, that is, from Republican to Democratic or vice-versa.

Testifying

Presenting testimony at a committee hearing for a bill often resembles a situation in which adversaries and advocates are pressing their points.

For the testifier, it is lobbying, argument, and negotiation. For the committee, it is an interview in which each member tries to acquire as much information as possible on disputed points. Rather than a compromise, however, the ultimate decision usually favors the advocate or the adversary.

In preparing testimony, ask yourself three questions:

1. Is the bill simple, without strong or effective opposition?
2. Is the bill complex?
3. Does the bill have strong or effective opposition?

If the bill is simple and has no strong or effective opposition, your testimony will be a straightforward explanation of the bill and the rationale for it. The four kinds of argument on pages 153–156 can provide one or more points for your rationale.

If your bill is complex or if it has strong or effective opposition, then your presentation is a preparation for argument and strategy. You can prepare a written statement, a formal argument, usually about five to ten, typed, single-spaced pages. Make a copy for each member of the committee, the staff, and any media persons present. However, don't read the argument. In testifying, you want to speak spontaneously, demonstrating your thorough preparation and grasp of the matter.

Prepare as you would for negotiation (Chapter 6); plan your lobbying tactics; analyze the adversaries' arguments in terms of the fallacies discussed above. Remember that your audience is the committee, not your adversary. You want a majority of the committee to vote for your side, so you should be aware of their past attitudes toward healthcare issues and the reasons any of them might have for adopting an adversarial position. A part of your argument should attempt to nullify or lessen those reasons as well as those of your stated adversaries. Emphasize any weaknesses in the adversaries' position and the strengths of your position. Because fiscal considerations cause concern, state realistically what the fiscal impact will be. Don't fudge your figures because you will be caught, thereby invalidating the rest of your testimony in many of the committee members' minds.

Another important factor in testifying is the visible presence of supporters of your stance. As soon as you know the date, time, and place of the hearing and your testimony, notify your healthcare organization and any other supportive group to arrange for a supporting delegation. Such visible support will impress the committee. However, the supporters should be polite and in no way disrupt the proceedings.

The following points should guide you to successful testimony:

1. Arrive early. You may need to complete some forms. Ask the secretary or the member of chairperson's staff.
2. Dress conservatively. Conservative dress implies respect for the committee and for legislative proceedings. It also suggests competence.
3. When called to testify, introduce yourself and identify whether you are speaking for yourself or representing your healthcare organization.
4. Present a clear, concise summary of your position and your rationale. Don't repeat yourself or talk long on any point.
5. Avoid technical language and visual aids. Any visuals should be transformed to figures or tables appended to your written testimony.
6. Confine your testimony to one or two major points. You will most likely have only 5 minutes to testify.
7. If you propose changes or additions, present them, typed, to the committee.
8. Be prepared to answer questions from the committee. Give direct, concise, informative answers. Remember, the purpose of the hearing is to gather information. Hostile reactions, bickering with committee members, or threatening them are totally out of place, no matter how hostile a question, a tone of voice, or a behavior might seem.
9. Upon completion of your testimony, hand your written testimony to the secretary or a staff member. Sometimes, you might wish to present this written testimony prior to the oral testimony. You risk, however, the committee's reading rather than listening attentively.
10. Express your appreciation to the committee and its staff for its time and thoughtful attention to your testimony.

If you are in charge of rounding up persons to testify, select persons who are knowledgeable, make a good impression, and speak clearly. Present these testifiers in a brief and orderly succession.

Whether you are testifying, supporting, or managing, be attentive to the adversaries and to any adverse criticism from the committee.

An Unusual Case History

Although most healthcare professionals think of lobbying as the process described in this chapter, it is important to remember that negotiation and communication are also parts of lobbying. Likewise, lobbying does not have to be confined to the legislature. You can lobby a regulatory agency or a court. A recent decision of the Missouri Supreme Court demonstrates this sophisticated form of lobbying.[4]

Two nurse practitioners, Suzanne Solari and Janis Burgess, were charged with practicing medicine without a license. The physicians with whom they worked were charged with aiding and abetting them. The County Circuit Court upheld the charges. However, the Missouri Supreme Court reversed the decision of the lower court. In arriving at their decision, the judges studied various documents as well as the statutes. Among those documents were over one hundred briefs submitted as "friend of the court" (amicus curiae), a usual practice to provide a court with additional information. Although far more formal and detailed, such briefs are not unlike the letter presented earlier in this chapter. In the Missouri case, the briefs detailed the historical development of nursing and the expanding role of nursing in delivering health care. The court recognized that the defendants were consistent with current practice and education of the profession in both Missouri and the United States and that such practice was consistent with the intent of the 1975 statute to make legal the expanded functions of nursing. In finding for the defendants, the court compared the number of briefs to a letter-writing campaign addressed to a legislature. The comparison is appropriate.

Summary

Lobbying is an intensive year-round activity. The lobbyist goes through a cycle of preparing, talking, writing, monitoring, evaluating, and preparing again. A lobbyist needs knowledge of the lines of power, the law, the legislative process, and the legislators. A lobbyist must know how to negotiate and how to use the media. A lobbyist spends the day touching bases to get or give information. It is a demanding yet exhilarating job. Although most health professionals will not become lobbyists, they need to know what lobbying involves because it is likely that they will participate in indirect lobby or committee hearings. Knowledge of lobbying will help them or their professional lobbyist to lobby more effectively.

Notes

[1] *The Washington Lobby*, 4th ed. (Washington DC: Congressional Quarterly, Inc.), p. 8.
[2] *The Washington Lobby*, p. 10.
[3] We thank J. E. Klagge and the Arizona Dept. of Transportation for permission to draw upon questions and adapt material from the booklets cited in the Reading List.
[4] Bullough, B. Legislative update. *Pediatric Nurse*, p. 162.

Suggestions for Additional Reading

de Kieffler, D. *How to lobby Congress*. New York: Dodd, Mead & Company, 1981.
Grimes, A. J. *A guide for providing scientific testimony*. Arlington, VA: The American Institute of Biological Sciences, 1977.
Klagge, J. E. *Issues and opportunities: Identification, prioritization, and implementation*. Phoenix: Arizona Department of Transportation, 1982.
Klagge, J. E. *Programmatic considerations in the legislative planning process*. Phoenix: Arizona Department of Transportation, 1982.
Murphy, T. *Pressure upon Congress: Legislation by lobby*. Woodbury, NY: Barrows Educational Series, Inc., 1973.
Smith, D. *In our own interest*. Seattle: Madrona Publishers, Inc., 1979.
The Washington Lobby, 4th ed. Washington, DC: The Congressional Quarterly, Inc., 1982.

Chapter 9

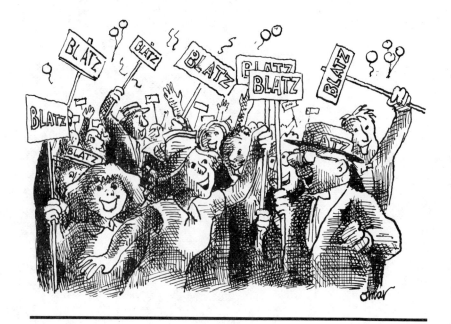

Political and Party Activity

In addition to involvement with one's professional organization or in direct or indirect lobbying activities, a health professional's involvement with specific political campaigns or in running for office can increase the political effectiveness of a health profession. Many health professionals have said to themselves, "*I* should run for state legislature" or "*I* could be a delegate." But they generally do not put the idea into action because the effort seems so vast. Instead of letting the idea go, the health professional might become involved in a campaign just to see what goes on. Through such involvement a person can become aware of the components of a campaign and the way they work. The person can also get to know legislators, party officials, and party workers, all of whom might become resource persons or workers for lobbying efforts or for one's own political campaign. Such involvement by health professionals can also build political IOUs and increase their expert power.

The purpose of this chapter, then, is to delineate the kinds of participation and the components of a campaign. Its intent is to demystify the process in order to encourage health professionals to participate in party activity or even to run for office.

Kinds of Participation

Participation occurs within an organizational framework. The major organizations, of course, are the Democrat and Republican parties. The term "Independent" signifies a disassociation with any party or its platform, but the candidate must still have an organization, one that frequently combines with those of other Independents in order to defray expenses and increase the effectiveness of volunteers.

One characteristic of political parties is the loose organization. In other words, one level of organization doesn't have control over any other level. For example, state officials are quite independent of the national organization, and precincts are quite independent of the county. However, there is a loose hierarchy (Figure 9.1) that can work together or not as need or desire might require. Figure 9.2 shows the relationship between state and national party organizations.

The political activities of all political parties, even Independents, are governed closely by state and federal law. Election law varies from state to state, but it controls qualifications to participate in party activities, procedures to get on the ballot, handling of finances, and organizational structure of the parties from precinct to state level. You can obtain these laws from local and state election officials, the League of Women Voters, or other political organizations.

Within this organizational framework are many kinds of political involvement. Deciding on your level of political involvement can be confusing. You need to consider your available time, your skills, and your personality. The levels of participation encompass mild interest, low-level participation, and high-level participation.

The State
State Chairperson
Other Officers
State Central Committee

The Counties
County Chairperson
Other Officers
County Central Committee

The Precincts/Wards
Precinct Captain
Precinct Committeepersons

Figure 9.1. *Political party organization*

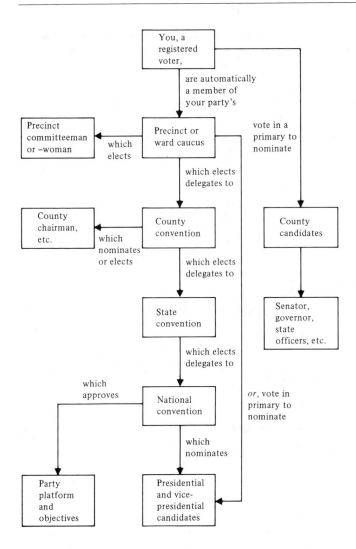

Figure 9.2. *The hierarchy of a typical political party*

Source: From *The American Political Process.* 2nd edition, by Charles R. Adrian and Charles Press. Copyright © 1970 by McGraw-Hill Book Company. Used with permission of McGraw-Hill Book Company. [Based on data from the Committee on Political Education, Labor and Politics. AFL-CIO, Washington, D.C. 19601.

Mild interest

This level of participation encompasses those health professionals whose interest in national, state, and local political news leads them to watch television, read a newspaper, listen to the radio, or participate in their professional organizations. The greater their intake, the more likely they are to vote, to display a bumper sticker, to wear a campaign button, to attempt to sway another persons's vote, to initiate political discussions, or to contribute money to a campaign.

Low-level participation

The health professional who participates at a low level of political activity is willing to call or write a legislator or agency official, attend a hearing or political meeting, or make a few telephone calls now and then.

High-level participation

The various activities of high-level participation range from the occasional to the constant. However, they all involve increased time, effort, and commitment.

People participating at this level become actively involved in a political party, attend strategy meetings, and contribute time and energy to a political campaign. They might not only contribute their own money to a political venture but also solicit political funds. Finally, a highly motivated individual will actually run for an office and upon election work with dedication.

Most health professionals participate at the levels of mild interest or low activity. However, more healthcare professionals need to become involved at the high level of activity. Many health professionals have the talents and assets to participate successfully in political campaigns or to run for political office. These individuals need to be identified and then encouraged and supported because their knowledge of the healthcare costs to the consumer, of the internal functions of our healthcare system, and of their professions make them valuable internal advocates. Having more internal advocates within the legislative and executive branches on the state and national levels is becoming increasingly necessary in that these branches are facing, with increasing frequency, decisions about health care.

Senator Lindeman—high-level involvement

Senator Anne Lindeman's career exemplifies the process of mild interest leading to participation to high-level involvement. Her career also illustrates that healthcare professionals have a place in legislatures.

After graduating as an R.N. from Memorial Hospital School of Nursing in South Bend, Indiana, Senator Lindeman married Robert Lindeman, an Air Force Lieutenant. Widowed and left with a 5-year-old, a 3-year-old, and a newborn, she sought a part-time position in nursing. In 1962, however, time-sharing had yet to be considered.

Unable to find a part-time nursing position, Senator Lindeman drew upon her interest in politics—an interest stimulated by her high school government teacher. She began working with a Phoenix Young Republican, now known as U.S. Senator Barry Goldwater. As she became involved, her high school interest rekindled, and she began her upward progress through party ranks, beginning as a deputy registrar, moving to precinct committeewoman, and then to district chairwoman. She also took a part-time position as secretary to a state senator.

When in 1972 there was an open seat (no incumbent) in her district, she decided to run for state representative and won. As a member of the Arizona House of Representatives from 1972 to 1976, she served on the following committees: Health, Education (as Vice-Chairperson), Government Operations, and Appropriations.

In 1976, she ran successfully for state senator. Presently a member of the state Senate, she is serving her fifth term. She has served and is serving on the following committees:

Majority Whip, 1983–1984
Senate Parliamentarian, 1979–1984
Education, Chairperson, 1979–1984
Appropriations, 1979–1984; Subcommittee Chairperson, 1981–1984; Vice-Chairperson, 1983–1984
Government, 1977–1982
Rules, 1979–1982
Commerce and Labor, 1983–1984
Health, Welfare, and Aging, 1977–1984
Legislative Council, 1981–1984

Joint Legislative Budget Committee, 1983–1984
Joint Legislative Reapportionment Committee, 1981

In addition to Senator Lindeman's considerable legislative responsibilities, she involves herself in various community committees. In 1982 she received the National Republican Legislator of the Year Award from the National Republican Legislators Association. Since 1978, she has been an active member of the National Conference of State Legislators. In the past few years, the number of registered nurses in the state legislatures has increased. They have created a subgroup, of which Senator Lindeman is a member, within the National Conference of State Legislators.

In response to queries about the compatibility of legislative activity and health care, Senator Lindeman has suggested that healthcare professionals should be more involved in the political process because general health bills have an impact on all professionals. She believes that healthcare professionals need to have knowledge of healthcare issues in general rather than limiting themselves to their particular area of health care. Health professionals should become involved on the grass-roots level and educate themselves in the political process, moving upward as they desire to city, county, state, or federal levels. According to Senator Lindeman, it is important to identify one's elected officials and become familiar with their stands on issues.

Executive branch involvement

The legislature is not the only place for involvement. In the 1984 race for secretary of state of Oregon, the state's second highest office, two of the three candidates had special interests in healthcare as well as backgrounds in legislative office. Barbara Roberts,[1] the successful candidate, had been a state representative since 1980 and majority leader from 1982 to 1984. In earlier years, she had been a volunteer lobbyist for handicapped children and a member of the State Advisory Board for Emotionally Handicapped Children. She had also served with the Woodland Park Hospital Board and the Mt. Hood Community Mental Health Center.

Donna Zajonic[2] was also a state representative from 1980 to 1984. During this time, she served with distinction on the state committees for mental health, economic development, and urban development. Prior to her legislative experience, she had received her B.S. in nursing from the University of Missouri and practiced mental health nursing from 1973 to 1980.

Rep. Zajonic believes that the 1980s will make new demands on health care. More agencies and healthcare providers work with needy people. The funding must stretch farther among an increasing number of agencies and providers. Cost containment is a concern. Decisions about ethics and technology in health care will occur. Hence, it is vital, she believes, for nurses to become politically active. She has found that her best assets as a politician are her nursing skills: the training and ability to work with people and the good problem-solving skills nurses usually have. For both Donna Zajonic and Barbara Roberts, excutive branch involvement was desirable.

Summary

Presently, politicians are struggling with healthcare cost containment; consequently, the professional groups need to take a hard look at cost effectiveness. They cannot just protect their turf. Furthermore, they need to become more proactive rather than reactive. There is a need to identify alternatives to problems and not just say, "No, it won't work." Since health care in the 1980s and 1990s will be increasingly in the political limelight, we need more healthcare professionals seeking political office. Judy Buckalew, special assistant to President Reagan for public liaison, focusing on health and social service issues, stated, "It is gratifying to me . . . to watch [nurses] become excited about the information I'm giving them and about becoming involved in the policymaking process."[2] Such excitement extends to most healthcare professionals. Once they are aware of the political process and the effects that their participation can have, most health professionals are eager to begin.

Components of a Campaign

Many potential office seekers are hesitant because they do not know enough about a political campaign. A political campaign involves setting up the organization and planning and implementing drives for registering voters, getting the vote out, recruiting volunteers, recruiting directors of other projects, and raising funds. Although the process is usually plan, recruit volunteers, and implement, this section will present the planning and implementing of an activity together to provide a usable overview.

The organization

The major positions in a political campaign are the campaign manager, the director for registering voters, the director for getting out the vote, the director for recruiting volunteers, the director for raising funds, and the treasurer. These people and the candidate constitute a committee for the overall planning of the campaign. The campaign manager acts as liaison between the candidate and directors, coordinates the main components, attends meetings and public appearances, solicits large contributors (when appropriate), and develops literature and letters.

Each project director will have a steering committee composed of people in charge of specific activities. This committee will devise plans and means of implementing them.

Registering voters

To plan a voter registration drive, the project director selects four people to head four areas: what to do, where to do it, when to do it, and who will do it.

The "what" person researches election laws and procedures, obtains voter registration lists, keeps in touch with election officials, and devises the procedure for registering voters.

The "where" person identifies areas with high percentages of unregistered voters who are likely to support health issues. Such targeting allows concentration of effort where such effort is most likely to produce results. Election offices will supply numbers or percentages of registered voters, precinct by precinct. Street, or walking, lists are available at many election offices or at the state headquarters of the party. The "where" person then confers with the committee to set the registration goal for each targeted precinct. Registering 50 percent of the nonregistered residents would be a successful drive.

The basic methods of voter registration vary from state to state. The five usual procedures for registration are deputy registration, postcard registration, branch registration, centralized registration, and election-day registration. *Deputy registration* allows volunteers, after a short class on their duties, to be officially deputized to register voters by going to their homes, places of employment, or other sites. Some states may require deputies to work in pairs: one Democrat and one Republican. *Postcard registration* allows volunteers to be roving registrars signing people up on the spot. The forms can then be mailed or delivered to the election office. The system of *branch registration* sets up sites such as bank or state offices as registration centers on certain days. The designation of branch sites varies according to each state. The *centralized registration* requires one location, usually the city hall or the courthouse, and generally limits registration to regular business hours. Finally, *election-day registration* is a system that allows registration of new voters on election day.

Based on the method that the state permits, the "where" person would identify walking areas, permitted branch sites, place of central registration, or voting sites.

The "when" person, considering registration deadlines, plots likely times for canvassing for each precinct. Party headquarters will often have lists showing occupants of residences. Inquiries of persons familiar with various precincts will also elicit useful information.

The "who" person, using the what, where, and when information, identifies recruiters of volunteers from among party workers and supporting organizations. This person also supplies the recruiters with specific, printed information about what to do and where and when to do it. Each volunteer will receive this information. The "who" person provides registration kits and assists recruiters with instructing the volunteers. A registration kit will usually contain, depending on the type of registration permitted, the following items:

1. summary of registration laws, requirements, and procedures
2. registration forms
3. street, or walking, list
4. precinct or area map
5. name tag
6. information to use when talking with potential registrants

A combination of mailing and telephoning works best for recruiting volunteers. The mailing should contain a fact sheet presenting the reasons for the drive, the goal, the number of volunteers needed, a delineation of duties, and the available areas and times. Times should be blocks of 2 to 4 hours. Allowing time for receipt, the recruiters call the prospective volunteers to solicit their time and energy. The recruiter should answer any questions, stress the small amount of time involved, and assure a companion volunteer or transportation, if necessary.

When the volunteers have completed their assignments, they should report to their recruiter. The recruiter, "who" person, and entire committee should warmly thank the volunteers for their efforts. A handwritten thank-you should follow. A party for the volunteers upon completion of the drive is appropriate.

The "who" person should keep a list of the volunteers' names, addresses, telephone numbers, and dates and hours worked, forwarding a copy to the central files.

Getting out the vote

The project director will oversee the printing of material that explains the candidate's stance on selected issues, that states where and when to vote, and that stresses the importance of voting. This material should be mailed a week before the election.

To recruit volunteers for addressing, stuffing, and stamping, the project director relies on the central file. However, in recruiting for telephone reminders the evening before and the day of the election, the project director can supplement with the volunteers who registered the new voters. A personal reminder from a person previously encountered is a stronger impetus than is a reminder from a stranger.

The project director will also need volunteers to baby-sit and to provide transportation. The calling volunteer should ask whether the voter needs either or both of these services, arrange a time, and pass the information to the project director. The project director should, in turn, pass the information to the person in charge of the needed service.

Recruiting volunteers

As described above, mailings plus telephoning is a good method for recruiting volunteers. In addition, the party headquarters usually maintains a central file organized by precinct. Coffees and meetings of professional organizations are effective also. Current volunteers can have coffees or some similar gathering at which the guests meet the candidate or discuss issues of common concern. Toward the end of the gathering, the host, hostess, or other person presents the need for volunteer workers for the campaign of the attending candidate or of candidates who support the guests' views.

The presentation should explain the various views and options for service. At the end of the presentation, each guest receives a sheet that asks for name, address, and telephone number and lists the activities needing volunteers. The presenter asks the guests to complete the identification information so that they will receive thank-you notes for attending. The presenter then asks them to volunteer by marking the activities that they would be willing to do. At this point, the presenter stops talking and lets the silence hang, answering any questions directly and briefly. After the guests leave, the host or hostess checks to make sure everyone completed a sheet. If not, he or she fills one out so that everyone will receive a thank-you.

Recruiting should be a continuing activity. Relying on the same volunteers time after time will cause many of them to burn out. Constantly replenishing and enlarging the pool of volunteers lessens the amount of work any one person must do. Moreover, getting more people involved broadens the foundation of the campaign. Project directors should forward copies of their lists of volunteers to the central file for future reference.

Other campaign activities

Depending on the size of a campaign, the remaining activities can each have a project director, or one project director can manage several projects, excluding fund raising. The more prominent of these activities are:

1. petition drive
2. preparation for mailings
3. yard signs
4. phone books
5. literature
6. victory party
7. poll electioneering
8. public appearances
9. fund raising

Fund Raising

Fund raising is as essential to campaigns as are volunteers. Without either, a campaign usually cannot even get started. Money for reproducing voter lists, for file cards, for telephones, for printing literature, for stamps: the list seems endless. However, most people would rather do almost anything than ask people for money. So, how do you get people to volunteer? You plan! And after you plan, you recruit area directors to help you plan some more. A thoroughly planned fund-raising campaign tries to account for every possibility — from a master plan to the script for telephone calls and the cost of stamps. With thorough planning, potential volunteers will know precisely what they will need to do and how to do it. If they know, they are more likely to agree to help. If they don't know, their imaginations take over, creating "worst scenarios," and scare them away.

It is important to keep remembering that well-planned fund raisers work. Otherwise, the mailers, telephone calls, and invitations to events that we receive for various causes would stop coming. For political campaigns they work also. They work best with a plan. Consequently, this section delineates a master plan and its parts. If you are a candidate, the plan provides an outline of what your campaign can do. If you are a potential or actual volunteer, the plan provides a guide for what a particular activity might involve and some suggestions for doing it.

Master plan

The master plan delineates who will be in charge, what will be done, and when it will be done. The process of deciding these questions will often involve several brainstorming sessions and several detailed discussions. In the beginning, the brainstorming might involve only the candidate and campaign manager because they must first decide who will be in charge. Ideally, the director for fund raising should have the following attributes:

1. Time and energy to devote to the campaign
2. Knowledge about sources for contributions. The person could have directed or participated in fund raisers before or know someone who has. Particularly important is knowledge about potential large donors.

3. Political experience. Expertise is not necessary, but previous experience in campaigns helps the person select the right activity and the right volunteer at the right time.

Upon selecting a director, include the person in all planning sessions thereafter. In other words, let the director direct. Future planning sessions should make the following decisions:

1. people — who will direct what activities
2. lists and records — who will develop lists of potential donors and keep track of responses, and what kinds of lists and record keeping are necessary
3. events — what kind of events and when they should occur
4. direct mail — how much, what kind, and when
5. face-to-face solicitation for large donors — what activities will elicit the most money
6. repeat solicitation — what activities will encourage previous contributors again, and how these activities should coordinate with other events
7. thank-you's — what system will most speedily get thank-you notes for contributing time or money *and* for attending events into the mail.

When making the master plan, remember that the function of fund raising is to raise money. Do not combine a fund raiser with another type of activity.

People

In addition to the director, a fund raising campaign will need activity directors for specific activities such as record keeping and events. Depending on the number and size of the events, assistant activity directors may be necessary.

The activity directors should form a committee that meets regularly. The committee should develop a timetable based on the estimated expenses for the campaign. The committee should ask the campaign manager for this estimate, both a total and a monthly estimate for the entire campaign. This estimate should include election night parties and any post-election-day activities. In making the timetable, the committee should be aware that expenses are heavier toward the end of the campaign and schedule the activities accordingly.

As the expenses of the campaign come in, the director of fund raising and the committee meet to decide which activities are best suited to fill immediate and long-range needs. Because campaign expenses can only be estimated in the beginning, the committee will usually need to add or repeat activities as the campaign progresses.

The committee also develops a budget for the expenses of fund raising itself. Telephones, postage, printing, travel, staff, facilities, decorations, food, and so on must all have their costs — both estimated and actual — entered into the budget. It is especially important that a record of actual costs exists. From such records, the committee can select the most cost-effective activities for any necessary repetition and indicate them for the next campaign.

A coordinator for implementing the master schedule is essential. This person makes arrangements for the activities, coordinates volunteers, assigns tasks, and works with the volunteers to be certain that everything gets done. The coordinator puts the master plan into action and is responsible for its daily working.

Finally, the volunteers make the activities work. They work under the direction of the coordinator and the director of their particular activity. The coordinator assigns them to an activity and sees that they carry out the activity director's instructions. As long as volunteers have clear, detailed instructions and close supervision, they do not need experience. Because happy volunteers need a clear chain of command, changes of instruction or personnel must come from the proper source: The activity director instructs; the coordinator assigns and oversees. The coordinator may, of course, suggest instruction to the director, and the director may suggest assignments to the coordinator. But instructions and assignments should not conflict.

Lists and records

Gathering lists of potential contributors and determining what kind of records are necessary and how to keep them need attention at the very beginning of the campaign.

Contributors. Develop lists from any source, and keep developing them as the campaign progresses. The candidate and spouse should each compile a list. Anyone from any place or time is appropriate, ranging from high school to personal and professional associations to friends and relatives. Members of the fund-raising committee should do likewise. Other sources for lists are previous contributors to the candidate, party, and other causes. For example, if the candidate favors some environmental position as well as a position on health care, contributors to environmental causes are potential contributors to the candidate's campaign. Political action committees, organizations and associations, labor unions, and the like are also potential sources for contributions.

In compiling lists the object is not just potential contributors but *likely* ones. For whatever reason, is there a likelihood that the person or group will contribute? Does the person have strong feelings about an issue that the candidate supports? Is he or she a past contributor, familiar with the candidate, and financially able?

Records. Before setting up a contributors' file, check with the secretary of state or county election offices (see Appendix A), whichever is appropriate, to determine what information and amounts the election laws require you to report. Set up 4-by-6 or 5-by-7-inch cards accordingly. Include the name, address, home and business phones, source of name (for example director of fundraising, party list) and any other business or personal information that might be useful.

Order the names alphabetically, and color code the cards to indicate size and likelihood of a contribution. A small contribution, $15.00 or less, could be blue. A medium contribution, $16.00 to 99.00, could be green. A large, $100.00 or more, could be red. This code will be useful for the various events: It would be fruitless to invite a potential small contributor to a hundred-dollar-a-plate dinner and wasteful to invite a potential large contributor to a $10.00 fund raiser. A second color code could be yellow for known contributors to the candidate or party, purple for known contributors to other political causes, and black for potential contributors whose records are unknown. Such coding will ensure that known contributors receive solicitations early in the campaign.

If you have access to a computer, enter the information in a data base program. Computers are faster than files, and you can cross-reference in several ways. Several software firms have designed programs for campaigns. Investigate what is available since such a program could be well worth the expense; however, be sure it fits your needs.

Events

Events will probably comprise the major source of funds. However, careful planning and no spur-of-the-moment purchases are fundamental rules. It is all too easy to have the costs outweigh the profits. If you can keep costs to 15 to 20 percent of the profits, you have an excellent money-maker.

When selecting events, try to be creative but not outlandish for the area and crowd. You want them pleased, not appalled. Creativity should focus on drawing people to the event and pleasing them when they get there. Survey what the popular entertainments in the area are, and try to work up an event that would be compatible. Auctions, sales, socials, block parties; receptions in homes, museums, well-known homes; carnivals; picnics; concerts featuring local musicians; raffles; rallies; theme parties: these are only a few of the many possibilities. Ask what other candidates have done that people liked, and be sure to modify your activity in some way to avoid copy-catting.

Events don't have to involve hundreds of people. For potentially large contributors, smaller events allow more time with the candidate and give them their money's worth, so to speak. The candidate and hearing the candidate's views provide the focus, so if the candidate is present and you have planned well with a touch of creativity, the event will be successful. A local celebrity can sometimes provide additional drawing power.

Be creative with time, also. Think of mornings, noons, and afternoons as well as evenings. Inquire about other events that might conflict with the selected time. For example, Wednesday evenings often have lower attendance because many church activities occur at that time. (You might, then, consider linking your activity to one of those activities some Wednesday evening.)

In planning the activity, allow sufficient time to complete all the arrangements. You will need to decide when, where, how to do it, and who will be in charge. You will need volunteers to carry out the plans.

Once you have compiled your list of potential contributors, you can attend to invitations. Try to make the invitations suitable for the event and the guests. Tell something about the candidate, and be certain to display prominently the date, time, and place. Enclose a response card (Figure 9.3) and self-addressed envelope. Get them printed in sufficient time to mail them two weeks before the event. If the guests are numerous, hold an addressing bee: Six people addressing fifty envelopes is faster than one person doing three hundred. Remember to write the guest's name on the back of the response card to ensure that you know who is and who is not going to attend.

After sending the invitations, make arrangements for food and drink and for recording the responses: Who is coming, and how much was the contribution. Keep the cards in alphabetical order so that you can enter the contributions made at the door. Call or visit the guests after a week to encourage them to attend and to mail their contributions.

Direct mail

Direct mail needs careful thought and sparing use. It is expensive. You need to design the letter, envelope, and reply card and have them plus the return envelope printed. You will need postage for both envelopes (don't rely on the recipient's having a stamp handy). You might even want to enclose some additional campaign literature, which although already printed has its own costs. If you are careless about the weight of the outgoing material and exceed one ounce for first-class mail, your postage increases.

To plan a direct mail campaign, you first need to compose the letter and decide who will sign it. The letter should sell the candidate — goals,

---

Reception for J. Doe, May 16, 1984
3:00 p.m. Civic Center

Yes, I plan to attend_____

No, I cannot attend_____

I enclose a contribution of: $15 $25 $50 $75   Other:_____

Figure 9.3. *Sample response card*

personal and professional experience, previous political experience, achievements, and so on. If the list is long, put it on a separate page — like a résumé — and devote the letter to the candidate's goals, citing a few items from the list to demonstrate experience. A good letter should not exceed two pages. Because recipients tend to skim the first and last pages of a letter then read the signature and any P.S., they tend to overlook the middle pages. State the request for a contribution in both the first and last paragraphs. Tell how the money will be used. Any P.S. should point out something additional that emphasizes the need for money and provides an interesting point. Have only one person sign the letter. If you wish, the letter can display other names at the side or bottom along with each person's campaign position and business affiliation.

Next decide whether to use first-class or third-class mail. The return envelope should always be first-class — you want the money quickly, and contributors do not like to mail money third-class. Third-class mail takes about 10 to 15 days longer than first-class.

The appearance should be personal. Avoid metered envelopes. Use, instead, commemorative or unusual stamps to catch the recipient's eye. Address the envelopes by hand. Hold several addressing parties if the mailing list is large. Doing a test-run first with a smaller list can give you some idea how well everything might work. If the response is poor, consider scrapping the campaign or reworking the letter.

A less expensive way to handle direct mail is to call first. Many local campaigns use this tactic to reduce expenses. Callers should state their own names, the name of the candidate they are working for, the office the candidate is running for, and the need for money. Then the caller should ask for a contribution: "Would you please contribute to John Doe's campaign?" If the person says no, ask if he or she would like some literature about the candidate. If the request for a contribution elicits a yes, ask whether the person would contribute $15, $25, $50, or more. Most people, after committing themselves, will follow through. If not, a "did you receive?" call can pinpoint the difficulty. At all times, be gracious and pleasant. Try to sound like you are calling a friend for some help. And be prepared to chat a few minutes if the recipient has questions, is undecided, or sounds friendly. Remember, no matter what the immediate response is, the person is a voter, and abruptness or rudeness can leave hostile feelings about the candidate.

Because many people are offended by calls soliciting money, it is a good idea to ask whether the call is interrupting dinner or some other activity. If so, ask whether you may call at some specific time. Name the time so that the recipient can say yes or no or name a different time. If the response is tomorrow, ask when would be a good time. Try to be as courteous to this stranger as you would be to a colleague.

If the direct mailing is large enough to make premailing calls out of the question, you might consider having an expert design and compose the letter. Public relations firms, advertising agencies, mailing services, printers, or managers of other campaigns can provide names of such professionals or may have such professionals on their staffs.

Whether or not you use a direct mail campaign, be sure to ask for contributions, stating the mailing address and name of treasurer, on all printed campaign material. Although responses from these are small, the request adds little to the printing cost and keeps the need for money apparent.

Face-to-face solicitation

A campaign targeted toward large contributors is essential because the greater portion of early campaign money comes from them. A face-to-face meeting is far more successful with such contributors than are mailings or telephone calls.

The bulk of such solicitation falls to the candidate. Hence, the candidate should rehearse and rehearse some more, role playing with the fund-raising committee and with persons who will ask penetrating questions. The candidate must appear relaxed, confident, and knowledgeable.

To tailor the request to each potential contributor, the candidate will need to know the following information about the contributor:

1. *What has the person or business contributed in past campaigns?* Tailor your request to this figure, perhaps a bit higher to allow the person to set the figure.

2. *Are there any mutual friends or friends of friends that the candidate can use as a reference?* Such a reference often increases the candidate's credibility. If the name is a friend of a friend, the candidate should meet the person, even if the meeting is just a 15-minute coffee break, so that the reference will not sound spurious should the contributor ask, "Well, how *is* Jane? Haven't seen her for a while."

3. *What approach does the potential contributor prefer?* Some *do* prefer a phone call; others don't like such calls during business hours. Some want a direct approach; others need a bit of stroking. Whatever you do, telephone first for an appointment. In general, keep the presentation to 5 minutes in length. The other information will come out as the person asks questions. The candidate should take along a variation of the media kit (see Chapter 11). This "contributor kit" might have an outline of the campaign, the intended literature — including the candidate's résumé — samples of buttons and bumper stickers, a list of fund-raising activities, and so on. Ask for suggestions. Many people like to give advice, and incorporating suggestions gives the contributor some vested interest in the running of the campaign without the candidate's giving anything away.

Once the candidate and contributor meet, the candidate should be alert for personal, professional, and political interests of the contributor. Incorporating those interests into the discussion of the campaign usually increases the contributor's interest.

Reserve asking for the contribution until the end of the visit. Be alert to signs that the conversation is winding down. At that time, take the cue and ask *directly* for a contribution of X dollars, a check *now* for X dollars. Then wait! Give the donor time to think. Don't be embarrassed by silence. The person has the necessary information. Burbling on, repeating things already said, implies embarrassment and uncertainty and softens the request. Just let the question hang in the air until the person responds. Silence has its own pressure.

Once the person responds, conclude the visit quickly. Thank the person for the contribution and/or time. Indicate that suggestions are welcome at any time. Ask permission to get in touch with the person later in the campaign if the person hasn't already revealed this information. This request is essential because most large contributors will contribute twice to a campaign. Furthermore, if the person didn't contribute this time, he or she might do so later.

Thank-you notes

Every contribution, every expenditure of time, and every attendance at any event needs *immediate* acknowledgement. Thank the person for the contribution and/or time. A face-to-face thank-you will *not* replace a written thank-you.

The thank-you notes should be personal. Handwrite and stamp them. The candidate should write the thank-you notes to the people whom the candidate has visited. The others can be handled by committee over the signature of the director of fund raising. If the event was especially large, a duplicated handwritten note is acceptable *only* if the printing is excellent.

Resolicitation

Indicate on the contributor's card whether or not the contributor has agreed to future communication. If appropriate, indicate "don't know." Add to the contributor's card any interests of the contributor or family: They could provide an opportunity later in the campaign to continue or improve the relationship. This awareness permits the candidate and campaign workers to become resource persons for the contributors' interests by sharing information about any upcoming event related to the interest. The event or information does not need to be campaign related. Finally, never hesitate to resolicit large donors. They will be the mainstay of the campaign. A pleasant request with an explanation of need will elicit a yes or no. The contributor will not turn into an ogre and gobble you up.

Control of funds

A primary rule of fund raising concerns handling money: Those who bring in the money do not spend it. All funds should go to a designated person. Check the election laws to determine whether this person needs a specific title such as treasurer.

All disbursements of funds should be made by check. The check and check stub should indicate what the expense was. The check should also have two signatures. The designated signers should be persons who are available on a daily basis. It is also wise to have a third designated signer in case someone is out of town.

The treasurer should have a calendar of estimated and planned expenses and of estimated income. As the estimated income becomes reality, the treasurer needs to make a list of the names of each contributor as well as amount of contribution. A copy of the list goes daily to the person keeping the contributors' card file.

Summary

Health care will continue to be an issue in the political arena, so healthcare professionals need to increase their political participation or begin to participate. The more health professionals who participate in the campaigns of candidates who are supportive of their views, the more direction they can have in their professions. They can increase their expert power and that of their professions. Participation on a small scale can lead to greater participation. Those persons who would like to run for office need encouragement.

The outline presented here of participation and campaigns is applicable to healthcare organizations as well as to the individual healthcare professional. Organizations can supply volunteers as well as contributions. They can conduct their own voter-registration drives and get-out-the-vote projects for healthcare issues. They can support those candidates favorable to the position and philosophy of the organization. The choices for healthcare professionals and their organizations are several. Knowing the components of a campaign enables them to choose the activities compatible with their time, energy, and skills to achieve successful results.

Notes

[1] N. Paulus, Secretary of State, Oregon, *The Official 1984 General Election Voters' Pamphlet*, Salem, OR 1984.
[2] Oregon nurse seeks second highest elective office in state. *The political nurse*, 1984, 4(3) 1–2.
[3] K. Morrisey, Spokeswoman in the White House, *Nursing and health care*, March 1984, p. 141.

Suggestions for Additional Reading

Agranoff, R. *The Management of election campaigns*. Boston: Holbrook Press, Inc., 1976.
Archer, S. E., and Goehner, D. A. Acquiring political clout: Guideline for nurse administrators. *Journal of Nursing Administration*, 1981, *11*, 49–55.

Archer, S. E., and Goehner, D. A. *Nurses: A political force.* Monterey, CA: Wadsworth Health Science Division, 1982.

Bagwell, M. Motivating nurses to be politically aware. *Nursing Leadership*, 1980, 3, 4-6.

DeLoughery, G. L., and Gebbie, K. M. *Political dynamics: Impact on nurses and nursing.* St. Louis: Mosby Co., 1975.

Ehrenhalt, A. The Fuller Brush approach to House campaigns. *The Congressional Quarterly, Inc.*, July 17, 1982, p. 1743.

Federal Elections Commission. *Federal election campaign laws.* Washington, DC: Government Printing Office, 1980.

Grissum, M., and Spengler, C. *Woman power and health care.* Boston: Little, Brown and Company, 1976.

Kalisch, B. J., and Kalisch, P. A. A discourse on the politics of nursing. *Journal of Nursing Administration*, 1976, 6, 29-34.

Kalisch, B. J., and Kalisch, P. A. *Politics of nursing.* Philadelphia: J. B. Lippincott Co., 1982.

Kayden, X. *Campaign organization.* Lexington, MA: D.C. Heath and Company, 1978.

Kelly, L. Y. *Dimensions of professional nursing,* 4th ed. New York: Macmillan Publishing Company, 1981.

Morris, D., and Hess, K. *Neighborhood power.* Boston: Beacon Press, 1975.

Mullane, M. F. Nursing care and the political arena. *Nursing Outlook*, 1975, *11*, 699-701.

National Education Association. NEA series in practical politics. Urbana, IL: NEA, n.d.

Roper, W. *Winning politics.* Radnor, PA: Chilton Book Co., 1978.

Stevens, B. J. Power and politics for the nurse executive. *Nursing and Health Care*, 1980, *1*, 208-212.

Wasserman, G. *The basics of American politics.* Boston: Little, Brown and Company, 1982.

Unit III

Increasing Political Clout

In Unit I you learned the fundamentals of power at work, the intent of the various kinds of law that shape political action, the boundaries that identify the various political players, and the structure and process of the legislative arena. In Unit II, you learned many of the plays that help to clear the path to the end zone, the achievement of your political goals and objectives. Awareness of the needs, motives, contexts, and constraints that limit both other players and yourself enable you to gain more yardage than you lose. Such awareness facilitates your application of the guidelines and formats for communicating with legislators and for effecting a lobbying campaign. As with Anne Lindeman, Donna Zajonic, Jay Goodfarb, and Judy Buckalew, whose mild interests in political action led to their high-level involvement, you, too, might decide to apply your increased political knowledge, awareness, and skills to party activity. Whether as a volunteer worker or a candidate, you can expand your political network through your co-workers and the constituents you meet.

Such involvement is certainly one way of increasing your political clout.

Unit III presents other means of increasing political clout. Networks, coalitions, political action committees (PACs), and use of the media are becoming essential plays for the playbook because the trend of the 1980s is the increasing politicization of health care. Consequently, health professionals need to become political professionals as well. Healthcare professionals need to network within their ranks to unify their goals and objectives. They need to network with those in other healthcare professions to clarify issues and eliminate misunderstanding. They need to create coalitions to work for common goals or to share resources by combining compatible goals. Finally, they need to become skilled in using the media as a resource: a source of information and a means of getting their message to the public, and indirectly, to the legislators. In these ways, healthcare professionals and their organizations can increase their political clout in the increasingly political decades ahead. It is essential that they unify so that as teammates they can hear their combined voices calling the plays over the roar of the crowd and the yells from the opposing team.

Chapter 10

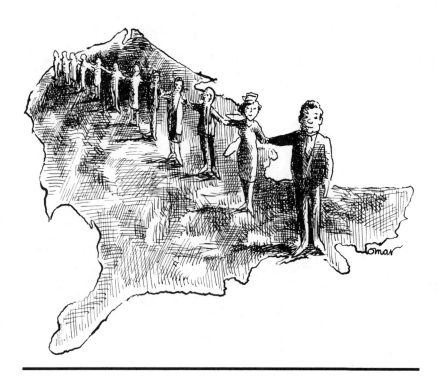

Networks, Coalitions, and Political Action Committees

In the last few years, several political forces other than the individual health professional and the individual healthcare organizations have arisen. The most common of these, and those having the highest visibility, are the PACs — the political action committees for various businesses and organizations, including the healthcare professions. Although lower in visibility, networks and coalitions can also be influential in the legislative arena and political campaigns. Indeed, their potential is becoming reality as healthcare professionals unite for a common cause. Each has its purpose, and there will be times when a healthcare organization can find them useful.

Because all these forms of political influence have advantages and disadvantages, this chapter describes what networks, coalitions, and PACs are and how they work so that healthcare professionals and their organizations can knowledgeably evaluate which kind is best for what situation. Such evaluation can increase healthcare professionals' participation in the political arena.

Networks

Networking is one response to the varied social issues and legislation that healthcare professions are increasingly facing. A network provides healthcare professionals and their organizations with formal channels for information, support, and strategy on a common issue. Not only is networking an excellent way of sharing information and resources, but it is also a rich source for new ideas and knowledge. A network can help local healthcare professionals become aware of, increase their knowledge of, and identify legislative issues on both state and national levels. It can not only provide information and knowledge to share with the members' organizations but also link healthcare professionals from different organizations and different states together in a forum for communication and action in politics.

For example, Delegate Marilyn Goldwater (D-Maryland) and Representative Mary Ann Arty (R-Pennsylvania) are forming a bipartisan network of nurses serving as state legislators and as policymakers in executive branches throughout the nation. As they state:

> There is strength in numbers; a group of well-focused, well-organized and well-connected individuals can work wonders through the political process. An idea proposed simultaneously in several states by a network of state legislators like ourselves quickly takes on the solidity and respectability of a trend. Trends get attention and often become law.[1]

How to form a network

To form a network, a committed core of health professionals should first survey healthcare organizations in their state for interest in networking. Second, they should formulate the process by which healthcare organizations would become members of a network and determine the members' financial responsibilities. Third, this committed core should determine the purpose and functions of the network.

In the first step, surveying the state to determine whether the professional organizations are interested in forming a network, the core people would talk with organizations for nurses, physical therapists, pharmacists, registered dietitians, occupational therapists, medical technologists, radiology technicians, respiratory therapists, audiologists, speech pathologists, and so on. The national and state healthcare organizations listed in Appendix B might be a beginning. They can provide information as well as names of people with whom to communicate.

Once one or two organizations indicate initial interest, then it is time for a written survey. The letter in Figure 10.1 is a sample of such a survey.

Professional Organization
Any Address
Any Town, U.S.A.

Dear President _____:

The healthcare climate in our nation has changed dramatically over the past few years. The registered dietitians are beginning to recognize the need to make decisions about their role in the healthcare delivery system, and since political decisions are crucial to these decisions, registered dietitians and other healthcare professionals must have input into their local and national legislatures. Because strong input is essential, it must be presented in a powerful voice by healthcare professionals who are united in a common purpose — to promote healthcare for the consumer.

Thus, the registered dietitians and nurses are forming a healthcare network in the state to provide some political expertise and are interested in inviting you to a meeting to discuss the purposes and functions of a network.

The meeting will be held on _____ at _____. If you need further information, please call me at 555-1529. Otherwise, we will be looking forward to meeting the representative from your group.

Sincerely,

Marvin Brown
MB:mmb

Figure 10.1. *Sample survey letter*

Once the meeting occurs, the participating healthcare organizations can assess whether there is sufficient interest in forming a network. If just three organizations express an interest, then a network is worthwhile. It might or might not expand rapidly because identifying new groups that could be effective takes time. Furthermore, the necessity of becoming politically active is a relatively new idea to many healthcare professionals and their professional organizations. As a result educating the members of the organizations to this need in the 1980s might be time-consuming.

The second step entails deciding on the type of membership, the organizational structure, and the processes of the network. Types of memberships might be voting and nonvoting memberships. The voting members could be those healthcare professionals whose organizations, associations, or services have appointed them to represent the organizations. Each organization would have one representative. The nonvoting members could be individual healthcare professionals who want to be active within the network, who support its purpose and functions, but who may not belong to a professional organization or a participating organization. The nonvoting member could pay $25.00 per year. The voting members' organizations could pay $50.00 per year dues and participate on the standing and adhoc committees.

The organizational structure could consist of an executive committee, public relations committee, health legislation committee, program committee, nominations committee, and any other committees the network might develop for specific healthcare issues. The executive committee might consist of the elected officers: president, vice-president, secretary, and treasurer. The public relations committee would be responsible for publicity, orientation, education, and recruitment of new members. The health legislation committee would monitor, critique, and report on bills. The program committee would plan and present programs and workshops. The nominations committee would prepare a slate of officers.

The organizational flow (see Figure 10.2) could be both an upward and a downward movement. One member could act as a legislative information reporter, whose function would be to relay information to legislators and to the executive committee — a liaison between the network and the legislature. Information would flow upward from the representatives and their organizations to the reporter, and downward from the reporter to the representatives and their organizations.

Once the structure develops, the third step is to determine the purpose and functions of the network. A usual purpose of a network is to provide healthcare professionals and health care organizations with a forum for discussion of issues concerning health care and a channel for information, support, and development of strategies pertaining to a common issue. Founding members, however, might want to broaden or narrow this purpose. A network usually has four functions: (1) informs and educates healthcare professionals about health legislation; (2) increases the political awareness of healthcare professionals; (3) encourages healthcare profession-

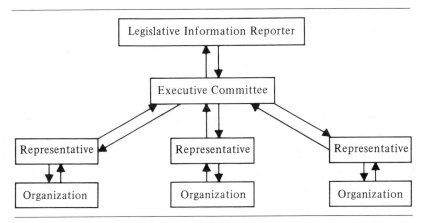

Figure 10.2. *Flow chart for a network*

als to participate in the legislative process; and (4) promotes and supports the advancement of health care through the legislative process.

To inform and educate healthcare professionals about health legislation, the network would schedule workshops to delineate and describe the legislative process, identify and clarify key issues that will affect healthcare, and explain any new legislation that affects the healthcare profession. This process would continue during the monthly meetings of the network so that the members could take this information back to their organizations. Discussions would also include all legislation that has an impact on health and the healthcare professions and that either has been introduced to the legislature or whose introduction is pending.

To increase the political awareness of healthcare professionals, the members would first identify what legislative district they live in and, in turn, have each member of their respective organizations also identify their districts and representatives. Then the network members communicate with their legislative representatives and encourage each of the individual members of their organization to do likewise. In essence, the network members are facilitators for getting the members of their organizations comfortable with the political process.

The Arizona Nursing Network, which coauthor Marilyn Bagwell designed and implemented in January 1978, in response to Senator Anne Lindeman's observation that nurses need to work together, has members from the network in each of the thirty legislative districts in Arizona. This representation enables the Arizona Nursing Network, which originally encompassed various nursing organizations but now includes other health-care organizations, to provide information to all the members of the legislature through a constituent. When the Arizona Nursing Network is seeking support in the legislature, it puts its telephone-communication tree into action (Figure 10.3).

The third function of the network, encouraging healthcare professionals to participate in the legislative process, is accomplished by having individuals and groups get in touch with their legislators and discuss the network's position on issues. The way to communicate with legislators was discussed in detail in earlier chapters. This type of systematic communication with legislators will increase the influence and effectiveness of the individual groups and the network because the legislators realize that the network can be a source of information about health care in a variety of settings as well as a power group that can influence a large number of voters.

The fourth function, promoting and supporting the advancement of health care through the legislative process, is accomplished not only by informing and educating but also by deciding on proactive and reactive strategies for influencing legislators. Since legislators make many decisions about a bill before its introduction in the legislature, healthcare professionals must provide information that goes into preparing bills. In providing this information, network members must be prepared to negotiate and compromise. They must analyze and interpret information concerning legislation and issue a network opinion. This opinion then goes to all organizations belonging to the network. When the network is ready for action in the legislature, it can hire a professional lobbyist or use a volunteer lobbyist.

In summary, then, a network is a speedy means of sharing health-care information and political expertise with many diverse healthcare organizations and professionals. It can provide a forum in which the diverse views of the diverse organizations can unite behind a common purpose. It can share the ideas and expertise necessary to devise and implement successful legislative strategy.

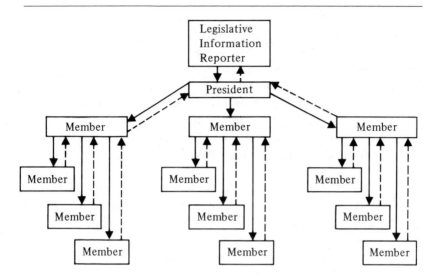

Note: All members have the home and work telephone numbers of the member immediately above and the members immediately below them on the tree to facilitate sending information up or down the tree.

Figure 10.3. *A portion of the communication tree for the Arizona Nursing Network*

Coalitions

Whereas networks offer a continuing alliance for the regular and sometimes speedy sharing of information and ideas, a coalition is a temporary alliance of groups for joint action. A coalition may be a result of networking: The member healthcare organizations temporarily take action together. However, a coalition can also include healthcare organizations that are not members of a network as well as civic organizations such as the Rotary Club, Lions, the League of Women Voters, and so on. When members of a coalition have divergent purposes and functions, cohesiveness derives from reciprocity. For example, a coalition's participating healthcare organizations would support certain legislative issues that members outside health care supported, in exchange for the support of those members on healthcare issues.

Building a coalition could increase the effectiveness of political action for healthcare organizations because it would increase their opportunities to communicate with legislators, it would expand the financial resources for conducting media campaigns, and the size of the coalition would attract the media's attention. In addition, the combination of staffs increases the number of persons available for various tasks. The increase in information gathering increases the effectiveness of each member of the coalition.

You could form a coalition in the following manner. Your healthcare network or your healthcare organization would identify its interests for the coming legislative session. Analysis of those broad-based, consumer health issues would indicate which organizations might be willing to form a coalition.

Upon identification of your prospective partners, your healthcare network or healthcare organization would then send out letters to each organization explaining that a particular healthcare issue might concern them. Identify these possible concerns. Ask these organizations to meet with your group to discuss the possibility of a coalition. Stress in your letter that their attendance is not a commitment but that you believe they can make a valuable contribution.

If the organizations indicate interest in exploring the idea, select a temporary committee to propose a structure and operation for the coalition. Of primary importance is the structure for decision making. The committee needs to determine an equitable means for determining positions and priorities. It needs criteria for establishing who will speak for the coalition. The committee would establish the following subcommittees: research; public information; finance; general administration, including office management; promotion of membership; political analysis; and voter registration.

At that time, schedule several future meetings. You should expect that the organizations will meet several times before they are willing to commit time and resources to the project. Once there is commitment, hold a general organizational meeting for adopting an organizational plan, choosing leaders, and beginning operation. Obtain commitments from the coalition members for contributions of staff, money, office space, telephones, and various miscellaneous expenses.

At this point, the coalition meetings would function like a network: giving and receiving information which representatives would take back to their organizations.

Success of a coalition depends on participation and knowledge. Representatives need to keep their organizations informed of and involved in the progress, activities, and tasks of the coalition. The representatives need to know the policies and programs of their organizations in order to share them with the coalition when necessary. These representatives also need to have a background adequate for dealing with the issue, and the time, energy, and interest to work with the coalition.

A coalition is truly a continuing negotiation. Every organization has its own interests and will be concerned that reciprocity might not occur. Negotiating fair shares for work, funds, space, and so on can be touchy. Each organization must feel that its participation is important to the effort and that its efforts are appreciated. As attention goes from one issue to another, organizations need assurance that their special concerns are receiving attention. As long as each organization feels that its rewards are worth the effort, the coalition will continue.

PACs

Political action committees (PACs) have a narrower purpose than that of either networks or coalitions: to endorse candidates for public office who support the concerns of the PACs and to contribute, when necessary, to the campaigns of those candidates. Through such endorsements and contributions, PACs enable individuals, businesses, and organizations to increase their access to elected officials.

Elected officials are now receiving considerable support from a diverse collection of PACs rather than a handful of "fat cats." However, the increase in support from PACs is itself causing concern. PACs have been extremely effective in gathering support for their concerns and stances on issues. Many people feel that PACs have been too effective, buying votes and support. As Archibald Cox, Chairman of Common Cause, stated:

> Over the years, Common Cause has kept a close watch on the relationship between PAC money received by congressional candidates and the votes these recipients cast on matters of importance to the PACs. Time

and time again, the studies show a close correlation between money received and votes favorable to PAC donors.

And the problem is getting worse. It appears that every group — except the people — now has a PAC. The number of special-interest PACs has skyrocketed, and the amount they are pouring into the political system has grown incredibly.[2]

Despite the negative reactions to PACs and the potential for limitations on their activities and contributions, healthcare professionals should know what PACs are and how they work. Such knowledge will enable them to consider whether or not to establish a PAC if their organizations have none or none at a desired level of political activity. After all, PACs *are* effective. For those healthcare professionals whose organizations have PACs, such knowledge can facilitate effective use of those PACs and might encourage some health professionals to seek appointment to their PACs. Finally, many of the techniques and processes that PACs have developed are adaptable to the activities of networks, coalitions, and individual healthcare organizations.

Types of PACs

There are two kinds of PACs: the nonconnected PAC and the separate segregated fund (SSF). The nonconnected PAC is neither connected to nor sponsored by a corporation or labor organization. However, it sometimes has a nonlabor and noncorporate sponsor, such as a partnership or an unincorporated membership organization. The SSF *is* connected to a corporation or labor union. In fact, it stands as the political arm of such a group. The PACs of several healthcare organizations, such as N-CAP for the American Nurses Association, are SSFs under the classification of labor organizations. The PACs of some other healthcare organizations may be nonconnected.

The sources of operational expenses differ. SSFs receive all of their costs for administration and solicitation from the connected organization. Such contribution is not subject to the yearly limitation on contributions. Hence, all the money that SSFs raise can go to candidates that they endorse. Nonconnected committees, however, must themselves pay all their costs of administration and solicitation. Any support from a sponsor is a contribution subject to the yearly limits on contributions.

There are also differences in legal targets for solicitation. A non-connected PAC may legally solicit *any* individual, group, or committee for funds. However, the SSF may solicit only a specifically defined, restricted class of persons. These persons are, under the class of labor organizations, the members of the organization and their families. Only these people may legally receive solicitations at any time and partisan communication from the organization.

A final major difference between the nonconnected PACs and SSFs is the $1,000 threshold. Under the Federal Elections Campaign Act, a non-connected group becomes a PAC when it receives contributions or expends monies in amounts greater than $1,000. On the other hand, a SSF becomes a PAC as soon as its connected organization sets up the SSF. It has 10 days after that date to register with the Federal Elections Commission by filing a Statement of Organization. This form requests from the SSF its title, the name of its connected organization, the names of other SSFs associated with it, the name of the treasurer, and the bank account from which the SSF makes expenditures and to which it deposits contributions.

Differences concerning the internal affairs, kinds of contributions, and disbursements are thoroughly covered in the Federal Elections Commission (FEC) publications *Campaign Guide: For Nonconnected Committees* and *Campaign Guide: For Corporations and Labor Organizations*. The FEC will, upon request, send them to interested persons. See Appendix A under the National heading for the address and telephone number.

PACs may organize on the local, state, and federal levels. Only at the federal level must they report the activity of their bank accounts and their contributions and disbursements to the FEC. The local and state PACs are, however, subject to state laws. Local PACs are exceedingly rare.

If there are state and national PACs, each connected to the state and national associations of a healthcare organization, these PACs are careful not to infringe on each other's territory or to impose their views on each other. For example, if a national PAC wants to support an incumbent U.S. Senator's candidacy, it will first inquire of the state PAC whether the state PAC can support the national PAC's endorsement of the candidate. If the state PAC says, "No way! Senator Doe has done nothing here for the healthcare profession despite what he might say in Washington," the national PAC will withdraw and not make the endorsement. The reverse is also the case.

Functions of PACs

In general, PACs — whether nonconnected or SSF — have similar functions. They endorse candidates, actively campaign for candidates or issues, raise funds, and educate their memberships in the political process and healthcare issues. The purpose of this political activity is, of course, to develop political power by electing candidates who are favorable to the endorsing PAC's stance on the issues and to the profession that the PAC represents.

Endorsements. Endorsing candidates is the most visible function of PACs. The media reports such endorsements regularly. Although the process of reaching an endorsement is not visible, it consumes considerable time. It does, however, acquaint candidates with issues of concern to the PAC and the PAC with the candidates' stances on the issues. When acquainted with these stances, PACs have the options of endorsing one or more candidates for a particular office, or no candidates for that office, or distributing funds to endorsed candidates. PACs often adhere to the following order of priority for endorsements:

1. Incumbents who have proven themselves friends of the profession the PAC represents or health care in general and whose reelection chances are marginal. Such candidates will often merit early endorsement.
2. Pro-healthcare challengers who have a good chance of unseating an incumbent who has proven unfriendly to the concerns of the PAC or health care in general.
3. Elections in which propositions affecting health care or the health profession that the PAC represents are on the ballot.
4. Pro-healthcare candidates who have a good chance to win an open seat — one for which no incumbent is running.
5. Pro-healthcare incumbents who do not face a difficult reelection campaign.
6. Other candidates, who will receive consideration on a case-by-case basis.

Whether or not to grant endorsements in a primary election is usually determined on a case-by-case basis. For example, when the ultimate winner of a race will be decided in the primary and there is a clear interest in one candidate's success, a PAC will consider bypassing the usual procedure for endorsement (if necessary).

When considering a candidate for endorsement, PACs often use the following procedure:

1. review a questionnaire that the candidate has fully completed
2. conduct a personal interview
3. examine an incumbent's voting record
4. examine a nonincumbent's voting record should there be one (for example, if a representative is running for senate or a city councilman is running for representative)

Table 10.1 displays the timetable that the very successful NEA-PAC (National Education Association) uses to ensure that its council receives the necessary information in sufficient time to review the materials. The process requires 90 days unless extraordinary conditions prevail. NEA-PAC suggests that the timetable should be sufficiently flexible for adaptation to local situations.

The questionnaire usually queries the candidate about specific issues of concern to the health profession that the PAC represents and to health care in general. For example, "Do you believe that it is appropriate for Congress to attach obligations such as collective bargaining rights to the receipt of Federal funds? Please explain how your answer would differ if the obligation were for civil service rules." Or "What role should the government have in the provision of healthcare services?"

A cover letter (Figure 10.4) and self-addressed envelope accompany the questionnaire to encourage full responses and prompt return of the questionnaire.

PACs usually try to review every race in their jurisdiction. For example, national PACs review U.S. Senate and U.S. Representative races. State PACs review all races for the state legislature, and local PACs review local races pertinent to their specific interests. To help screen the possibilities, national PACs try to have a Congressional district coordinator (CDC) in every state, and state PACs several state district coordinators (SDCs) in every state. As they review the questionnaires from the candidates, the

Table 10.1. *NEA-PAC Model Endorsement Timetable*

Endorsement Day	Activity
Minus 90 days	Selection of Interview Team for each Congressional District
−85	Notification of state body and NEA of contact person for Interview Team
−75	Mailing of NEA Endorsement Packet . . . to Interview Teams
−70	Training of Interview Teams . . .
−60	Preparation and mailing of Mail Questionnaire and Cover Letter to candidates . . .
−50	Telephone follow-up to candidates to maximize return of Mail Questionnaires
−35	Pre-interview orientation session of Interview Team to review Mail Questionnaires, Legislative Program, Interview Documents, and schedule and logistics of interviewing.
−45 to −30	Interviewing of candidates . . .
−35 to −20	Preparation of Tally Form summarizing candidates' responses and other data (within 10 days following interview)
−10	Analysis and/or comparison of Tally Forms
0	Voting on endorsements (as prescribed by state body)
+3	Notification of state body of endorsements
+7	Notification of NEA by state body via official Concurrence Form . . .

council or board of trustees will query the CDCs or SDCs about the candidates from their states. Such queries may occur before or after the interview.

The interview teams travel to the candidate's state or district if the legislature is not in session. In general, however, there is no commonality among PACs for the place of interview or level of the team doing the interviewing. If a profession has a national PAC but no state PACs or only a few state PACs, national teams might interview the candidates for state races in those states lacking a state PAC.

Although the number of persons on an interview team might vary

Dear_____

Our association is considering the endorsement of a candidate for Congress from the _____District in the coming election.

To assist us in determining whom we endorse, we would appreciate your completing and returning the enclosed questionnaire. Please feel free to provide additional information you feel will be helpful.

After we have received your questionnaire, we would like to schedule an interview with you to explore in more depth your thinking on key issues. We will set up the interview at your convenience.

We hope you will be able to return the questionnaire by_____.
Many thanks for your cooperation.

Sincerely,

Interview Team Captain

P.S. If you have any questions, please call me at _____.

Figure 10.4. *NEA-PAC sample cover letter for questionnaire*

from PAC to PAC, four of those persons should have assigned roles for the interview. A team should include a host, a captain, a reporter, and a tracker. Trade-offs from interview to interview are fine as long as the persons have the qualities essential for each role.

The following description (from NEA-PAC) of the functions and identification of qualities of key members of a PAC interview team might encourage some healthcare professionals to seek appointment to their state or national PAC. This information can be adapted to other situations.

Functions and Qualities of An Interview Team

1. The host meets the candidates and ushers them to the interview team.
2. The captain chairs the interview, asks questions from the interview guides, and recognizes others who wish to comment or ask questions. The captain should be friendly, courteous, and neutral. If necessary, the captain interprets the questioning and supplies background information.

3. The reporter listens carefully and observes facial expressions and body language. (Does the candidate stiffen a bit at the mention of collective bargaining?) The reporter should ask no questions but should know the issues. The reporter should also have a good memory (observing precludes note taking) and be adept at summarizing.
4. The tracker steers the conversation back on track if it goes astray. This person keeps the interview moving in the proper channels and keeps track of time. However, the tracker should not stifle digressions that give insights into a candidate's thinking. For each comment, the tracker must receive the captain's recognition.

The team will often include representatives from other levels of PACs. For example, a national PAC team might include the PAC chair or a representative of each local PAC in the Congressional district. The CDC for the district might also attend. Ideally, the team should be representative of the constituency as to race, age, ethnicity, and sex.

Interview teams usually have a list of questions to ask a candidate. Figures 10.5 and 10.6 show the interview guides that N-CAP interview teams complete and forward to the board of trustees.

The following guidelines are those that NEA-PAC furnishes its interview teams. They provide additional information about the interviewing process.

Interview Guidelines

1. Hold a pre-interview meeting to orient the Team to the schedule and procedures of interviewing. This "rehearsal" is vital to insure a smooth interviewing process.
2. Interviewing a House or Senate candidate should be a "class" affair — one that will increase the candidate's respect for teachers [health professionals] and their political action programs. Pick a location that provides a good atmosphere for the interview — a committee room of the State Legislature or a hotel meeting room. Avoid the Association office unless it contains a full-fledged conference room.

Please rate your Congressman/Congresswoman/Senator

1. Do you consider_____(Name)_____ _____(District/State) accessible personally to discuss issues, votes, etc.?

    Usually   _____
    Sometimes _____
    Rarely   _____
    Not at all   _____

2. Is her/her legislative staff readily accessible to the nurses in his/her district?

    Always   _____
    Usually   _____
    Sometimes _____

3. Are the needs and interests of the SNA sought out on health matters by the Congressperson/Senator *early* in the legislative process?

    Often   _____
    Occasionally _____
    Never   _____

4. How does the candidate respond to the following questions?

    a. What role should the federal government play in the provision of healthcare services?

    b. What do you see as the biggest contributing factor to escalating health costs and how should this be curbed?

    c. Should nurses with advanced training or certification in special areas be eligible for direct reimbursement for services they are licensed to provide under State law?

    d. What is the nature of your commitment to the protection of the rights of organized labor? Do you believe those rights should be extended to public employees?

Figure 10.5. *N-CAP Interview guide and recommendation form for incumbents running for U.S. House/Senate (Continues on following page)*

e. What legislative and institutional changes are necessary to insure that women have equal access to the job market and are justly compensated for their work?

5. Do you hope to see him/her reelected?

Strongly yes   _____
No strong feelings   _____
Would prefer another candidate _____

6. Do you think this candidate should receive N-CAP endorsement?

Yes_____   No_____

If yes, what priority?

7. Are nurses working in this campaign?

If there are substantial reasons for N-CAP to stay out of this race, please so indicate.

Authorized signature_____

Position_____

Figure 10.5 *(Continued)*

---

3. The Captain should chair the meeting, and any other members of the team who desire to speak should be recognized by the Captain. The Captain should introduce other members of the Team at the beginning of the interview.

4. Set up a schedule of interviews and stick to it. Don't make candidates wait. Allow time after each interview for reviewing and writing comments. A full interview with post-interview discussion should run about 90 minutes.

5. Tape-record the sessions with the permission of the candidate — but allow off-the-record comments. Taping allows the Team to concentrate on questions and answers, not note taking. Transcribe the sessions and provide transcripts to each Team member — it's well worth the cost.

6. Allow the candidate time to deliver an opening statement if he or she desires.

_____

_____   _____
        (Name)   (District/State)

1) What is the candidate's experience in relation to health issues?

2) If he/she has been a member of the legislature, or other body, what was candidate's record on health and labor matters of interest to ANA/SNA?

3) How does the candidate respond to the following questions:

  a. What role should the federal government play in the provision of health care services?

  b. What do you see as the biggest contributing factor to escalating health costs and how should this be curbed?

  c. Should nurses with advanced training or certification in special areas be eligible for direct reimbursement for services they are licensed to provide under state law?

  d. What is the nature of your commitment to the protection of the rights of organized labor? Do you believe those rights should be extended to public employees?

  e. What legislature and institutional changes are necessary to insure that women have equal access to the job market and are justly compensated for their work?

4) Do you recommend endorsement of this candidate?

  Yes_____   No_____

  If yes, what is its priority?

5) Do you recommend another candidate for support?

6) Are nurses working in this campaign?

If there are substantial reasons for N-CAP to stay out of this race, please so indicate.

                          Authorized Signature_____
                          Position_____

_____

Figure 10.6. *N-CAP Interview guide and recommendation form for nonincumbents running for U.S. House/Senate*

7. Follow up on vague or incomplete answers. Pin candidates down. Paraphrase their answers to assure understanding ("Are you saying that you oppose . . .?").

8. Apply the same standards across the board. For example, use the same Team, Questionnaire, and Interview Document for interviewing all candidates. The easiest way to sell an endorsement is to observe a pure process.

"To sell an endorsement" means to convince the board of trustees to endorse a candidate. The data that an interview team elicits from a candidate comprise the means for doing so. After the interview, the team records the candidate's responses and sends them to the board along with a recommendation for endorsement or no endorsement. The N-Cap interview guides (Figures 10.5 and 10.6) include this information at the end of the forms.

If in the interview the candidate reveals misinformation or a lack of information about healthcare issues, follow up. Write a letter that politely corrects, clarifies, or informs. Or follow up with a personal visit if that is feasible. Sometimes several letters or visits might be necessary to make sure that the candidate clearly understands the profession's stance on an issue and the reasons for it.

In addition to the functions, qualities, and guidelines above, the following tips for interview teams and their individual members provide information that can make the interview go smoothly and elicit the desired information from the candidates. The tips also identify potential problems in the process and suggest solutions.

Tips for Interview Teams

1. Use the same interview team for all candidates for the same office. Although one tries to capture everything, there are nuances and fleeting impressions that frequently elude capture. The necessary ranking will be more useful coming from a team that has had the opportunity to compare and contrast all candidates. In other words, by seeing them all, the team will know which, if any, is best.

2. Have orientation sessions to familiarize all team members with their individual functions and the function of the interview.

Review issues and materials. Role play until everyone feels comfortable and confident.

3. Talk little. Remember, the team is interviewing, not being interviewed. Ask questions, paraphrase, provide background, and so on only to clarify, understand, and provide context. Be brief. Supply just enough to keep the candidates talking.

4. Tackle one interviewee at a time. Even though the team is exhausted, feeling short of time, and so forth, interviewing two or more candidates simultaneously or setting up a debate will defeat your purpose. First, the candidates may be less than honest or direct, and they have a better chance of avoiding being pinned down. Second, they may fall into campaign speech 83, paragraph 19, which will tell you little. Third, observation of reactions will tend to be ineffective with more than one person to observe.

5. If the candidate tries to interview you, return the question, "I was just going to ask you that very question." Or answer in one or two short sentences and conclude with a question of your own.

6. When the candidate has completed an answer, don't comment. Instead, ask another question.

7. Avoid clueing the candidate to the "best" answer. Keep words and phrases objective — no derogatory or laudatory words. Don't say what *you* think.

8. Be observant. Watch the candidate's facial expressions and body language. Listen carefully for tone of voice and judgmental words and phrases. Determine whether odd pauses are merely the manner of speech, a lack of information, or a hint of evasion.

9. Make the candidate comfortable. Offer coffee or some simple refreshment. Despite your personal preference, supply an ashtray. Remember you are after information. Smokers are often habituated to having a cigarette when they come upon a point they need to ponder. Deprivation makes them uncomfortable and can invite abrupt answers when you want elaboration.

10. Provide name plates for the table or wear name tags. Name plates are easier to read.

11. Be bipartisan. No matter how strongly you might feel about a topic, detach yourself. If necessary, pretend you are a scientist looking through a microscope at a very curious bit of life. You simply want to know how it works and why so that you can later describe it for your colleagues. In other words, look at the candidate's side of the matter to understand what that side is, what its sources, contexts, and constraints are so that you can determine what the implications are. A bipartisan approach can sometimes lead to surprising conclusions.
12. Save any commitment to the candidate until later. If you feel yourself warming to the candidate's views, remember that you have yet to discuss with your teammates whether the candidate really believes those statements. Remember, the candidate would like the PACs endorsement and money and will try to tell you what you want to hear.
13. Send *hand written* thank you's to the candidates interviewed.

Campaigning. PACs campaign in the manner of individual persons and healthcare organizations described in Chapter 9. They recruit volunteers for political campaigns of the candidates the PAC endorses. They train these volunteers for the tasks that the campaign managers have identified as being in need of volunteers. And they supervise those volunteers to be certain the tasks are done well and on time.

The volunteer bank should maintain a backlog of work so that volunteers who have made the effort to report will have constructive work to do. It is helpful to get the volunteers to commit themselves for 2 to 3 hours weekly or twice monthly and to report regularly at the stated times. In this way, the volunteers have a routine that they can work into their weekly or monthly schedule. Such a routine is often preferable to frantic, last-minute calls.

A card file of volunteers is also helpful. It could be set up alphabetically by district. Moreover, if several volunteers are employed by health agencies, e.g. hospitals, a file indexed by agency could also be useful.

Research is another part of the campaign process, as Chapter 9 described. PACs research a constituency in a manner similar to that of a candidate for office, as the following activities indicate.

Research to Increase Effectiveness

1. Identify targets for political action.
2. Identify the leaders and influential people in the area as well as establishments that provide good sites for literature.
3. Obtain precinct maps and the maps for state legislative districts and congressional districts.
4. Obtain a Precinct Locator from the elections office. From this document, PACs can determine the precinct for any address.
5. Prepare an election calendar for important dates in the election year.
6. Develop a demographic profile of the area using information from the U.S. Census Report.
7. If the PAC is an SSF, canvas the membership of the health association with which it is connected to develop a membership profile. If a nonconnected PAC has a sponsor, it could do likewise.
8. Establish a clipping program, similar to the one described in Chapter 11, to create files on incumbent office holders and announced candidates.

In campaigning, a PAC will work to get the members of the health organization to the polls to vote. It will, of course, encourage the members to vote for the candidates and issues that the PAC has endorsed.

Finally, PACs usually encourage the members to become involved in party affairs on their own. They recognize that the more of their members who become active in a party, the more opportunity the members have to achieve delegated power, enhance their expert power and that of their profession, and — perhaps — begin a foundation for traditional power.

Fund Raising. Fund raising will be little different from the description in Chapter 9. However, if the PAC is a SSF, the fund raising is restricted to members of the health organization it represents and to their families. If the PAC is nonconnected, the fund raising may solicit funds from anyone.

Education. PACs also try to educate people to the issues affecting health care and the health professions they represent. If an SSF, the PAC targets the members of its affiliated organization. If nonconnected, the PAC targets the public. They will identify and clarify the issues so that the targeted persons will understand the stances the PACs take and the endorsements they make.

SSFs assume that the better politically educated the members of their associations are, the more politically active they will become. They will volunteer, vote, and become active in their parties. Recently, healthcare PACs have been encouraging members of their associations to run for delegate to a national convention. They would like these members to become delegates in order to have as many healthcare professionals as possible serving as delegates to both the Republican and Democratic presidential conventions. Many delegates concerned about healthcare issues could strengthen or initiate healthcare planks in the platforms of the two parties.

Summary of PACs

PACs focus on electing those candidates who support their concerns and stances on issues. Their activities include interviewing, endorsing, contributing to campaigns, campaigning, fund raising, and educating. This narrow focus has made PACs extremely effective in their efforts. Despite some concern that they are too effective and some efforts to limit their activities, PACs are indeed an option for healthcare professionals to consider. Also, their techniques and processes are transferrable to other situations.

Summary

Networks, coalitions, and PACs are three means of increasing political clout. PACs can serve as the political action arm of a healthcare profession organization, as N-CAP does so successfully for the American Nurses Association, or they can be nonconnected entities working for the goals of one or more organizations. Networks can bring together healthcare professionals from different areas of the same profession, from different healthcare professions, or even from different states or parts of a state. Their functions are to gather and disseminate information, determine general goals and policy, educate the membership and the members of those organizations about the political process, healthcare issues, and legislative action, and to participate in the legislative process. Coalitions are temporary alliances of groups for joint action. Coalitions may derive from a network, occur when networks don't exist, or include organizations outside health care.

With networks, coalitions, and PACs forming and reforming among various healthcare organizations, the 1980s and probably 1990s will be years of alliances for effectiveness in the legislative areas. Knowing what kinds of alliances are possible and how these alliances work will enable healthcare professionals to select appropriate options and to contribute to successful legislative programs. The strength of the healthcare professionals will increase as they work together within their professions and with other health professions. A search for the common ground, rather than emphasis on differences, will provide the political effectiveness that the coming decades will require.

Notes

[1]Goldwater, M., and Arty, M. A. Nurse legislators build bi-partisan network. *The Political Nurse*, 1984, 4(3), 2–3.
[2]Political action committees — Pros and cons. *Consumers Digest*, 1983, Nov.–Dec., p. 24.

Suggestions for Additional Reading

A practical guide to coalition building. New York: Institute on Pluralism and Group Identity, 1976.
Archer, S. E., and Goehner, P. A. *Nurses: A political force.* Monterey, CA: Wadsworth Health Science Division, 1982.
American Association of University Women. *AAUW community action tool catalogue: Techniques and strategies for successful action programs.* North Carolina: AAUW, 1981.
Bagwell, M. The nursing network: A united front. *Nursing Leadership*, 1980, 2 (2), 5–8.
Bagwell, M. The politics of nursing. In Schoolcraft, V. (Ed.). *Community Health Nursing.* New York: John Wiley & Sons, 1984.

Federal Elections Commission. *Campaign Guide: For corporations and labor*. Washington, DC: FEC, 1983.

Federal Elections Commission. *Campaign Guide: For non-connected committees*. Washington, DC: FEC, 1983.

Federal Elections Commission. *Non-party political committees alphabetical index*. Washington, DC: FEC, 1984.

Federal Elections Commission. *Sponsor/Committee index*. Washington, DC: FEC, 1984.

Naisbett, J. *Megatrends*. New York: Warner Books, 1984.

National Education Association. *NEA series in practical politics*. Washington, DC: NEA, n.d.

National League for Nursing. *Public policy bulletin*. Washington, DC: NLN, 1982.

Nurse's Coalition for Action in Politics. *Time for nurses to make a difference through politics*. Washington, DC: N-CAP, 1981.

Puetz, B. F. Networking for nurses. Rockville, MD: Aspen Systems Corporation, 1983.

Smith, R. Pac-men: The new breed of influence peddlers. *Consumers Digest*, 1983 (Nov.–Dec.) pp. 23–24.

Wagner, P., and Smith, L. *The networking game*. Network Research, Inc.

Chapter 11

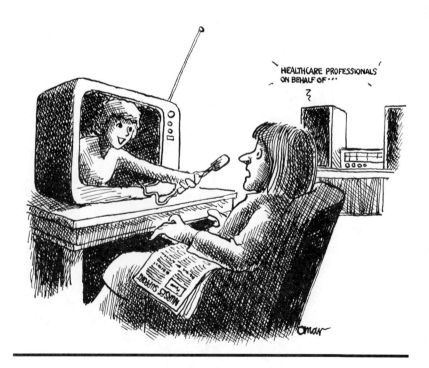

Media

For the average person in the United States, the major sources for political information are television, newspapers, radio, and magazines. Consequently, politically motivated health professionals should watch, read, and use the media for gathering and dispensing political information. Although each medium, and each outlet within each medium, has individual preferences and criteria, there are guidelines that can direct health professionals toward effective use of the media for political information.

Political information constitutes any information that healthcare professionals or their organizations dispense with the intent of aligning the media and their audiences (readers as well as viewers and listeners) with a particular viewpoint. *Direct information* influences an audience through facts, figures, reasoning, examples, situations, and the like. *Indirect information* influences through public service events, sponsorship of events, or human interest stories. Political information may work directly to recommend a particular stance on an issue, support for or opposition to a bill, initiative, or referendum, or support for a political candidate or event. It may also work indirectly to convey the responsibilities and expertise of the members of a particular health profession in order to create an understanding and positive impression. Such an indirect approach might later incline an audience to support particular political recommendations that the healthcare profession makes directly.

The indirect approach needs to be charted over time. It should make use of such media spots as public service announcements and programs, talk shows, personality spots, feature stories about local people and professions, human interest features in weekend magazine supplements in newspapers, and the like. By surveying the various media outlets in your

217

area, you can gather a list of possibilities that can provide a focus and goals for a long-range campaign. This indirect approach can help to build expert power in the minds of media people and their audiences.

Usually, however, most media campaigns are direct. There is an issue, a problem, a bill, a candidate needing support, clarification, or some political action *now*. Many national and state organizations have pamphlets giving hints, dos, and don'ts for working the direct approach with media people. If your organization has one, write for it. This guide will ensure that your approach is consistent with that of your state or national organization. For example, the American Nurses Association has a handy pamphlet, "Handbook for Political Media," which provides guidelines in very brief form. It is an excellent starting place and provided several categories and points for this chapter.

This chapter identifies the guidelines common to the literature and media professionals for a direct approach with the media and supplements them with points gained from personal experience. This information is flexible. You can adapt it to fit various personalities, outlets, and geographic areas. Local circumstances will dictate how much of the information is appropriate for your use.

Selectivity

Because you can use only so much information for political ends, selectivity is essential. Media people are inclined to place or follow up on (1) endorsements of candidates, (2) hard data concerning current healthcare issues that affect the public, (3) events that feature a candidate for office or a well-known elected official, or (4) other data and stories that currently interest the public or are important for the public well-being. Currency is vital. An article or news release pertaining to the status of minorities or women would have been current 3 years ago and will receive little more than a glance today. However, an article or release concerning containment of health costs is likely to receive an editor's attention because the public, health organizations, and governments are actively wrestling with the problem. Discussing an idea with a public service editor or feature editor may result in an angle that will appeal to or be important to the public. A human interest story or pictoral story could key to a news "peg" such as Senior Citizens Week or Health Awareness Week. Since media representatives are swamped with requests for coverage, they appreciate those persons and organizations who can select current information important to their respective audiences. You can help by attaching a note to an article or release or by personal communication. Sometimes explaining how your release relates to current concerns can help media people understand the importance of your news. Ideally, of course, the importance should be evident in the release.

One-Person Campaign

Individual communication with the media is frequently confined to letters to the editor and human interest stories keyed to a news peg because most health professionals lack the time to conduct a one-person media campaign. However, it is not impossible to do so on a small scale. In the course of 6 months or a year, depending on the size of a town, getting acquainted with the various editors and feature writers of a local newspaper or television station can provide you with ideas for stories and angles for releases. It can also establish you as a potential source when the editor or reporter needs health-related information.

To be effective in a one-person campaign, you need to remember that stories, releases, and remarks attributed to you will most likely identify your health profession. Such identification implies that you represent the members of your profession. Hence, you need to know the views and reasonings of your local, state, and national organizations. Keeping in close touch with these organizations can provide you with data that you might not have the time or the resources to obtain. If your one-person campaign is a dissenting voice, then make clear the issue(s) and reasons for dissent. Do not imply that you represent any other health professional or organization. Do be precise with facts and figures to support your view because those holding opposing views will be quick to argue forcibly for their own stance. Any errors or imprecision will weaken your case.

The guidelines for a one-person campaign are similar to those for an organizational campaign. The scale is merely smaller.

Organizational Campaign

An organization's effective political use of the media depends on its having a person who is willing to coordinate the collection and distribution of information. Responsibilities usually accompanying the position of such a media coordinator are the following duties: (1) researching; (2) establishing and maintaining organizational flow of information, including record keeping; (3) writing, speaking, listening, and responding; and (4) delegating responsibility.

Of these responsibilities, the essential ones are assigning responsibility, establishing and maintaining the flow of information, listening, and responding. If the media coordinator has limited time or is weak in skills such as researching, record keeping, writing, and speaking, then delegating them to persons who are effective in these areas is sensible. Such delegation also lessens the possibility of burnout.

Regardless which responsibilities the media coordinator retains or delegates, the following activities are essential to an effective media campaign:

1. Develop and maintain files
   a. media outlets
   b. releases circulated and covered
   c. media coverage of health care, healthcare professionals, and professions
   d. media inquiries
2. Write and distribute news releases
3. Establish a network among media representatives
4. Prepare oneself and others for interviews, participating in news conferences, responding as identified spokesperson
5. Communicate with local, state, or national organizations, as necessary, to
   a. gather data,
   b. ensure consistency,
   c. keep them informed of activities and issues covered by local, state, and national media.

Files

   Media Outlets. Develop a card file of the various media outlets that report health issues and the political activities of healthcare professionals and their organizations. Divide the file into kinds of outlets, and alphabetize the outlets by name within each division. Color code or name code the cards to ensure against misfiling. The card for each newspaper, magazine, journal, wire service, and radio and television station should have the following information:

1. *Name* of outlet.
2. *Telephone* number.
3. *Address,* including zip code.
4. *Schedule* of publication or airing: Daily, weekly, monthly, quarterly. Include specific day(s): for example, Weekly — Thursdays; Monthly — third week. For radio and television stations include the time: for example, Weekly — Thursdays — 7:30 P.M.
5. *Circulation.* Knowing the size of the readership or viewing audience can help to determine where to focus one's energies should time and assistance be limited.
6. *Type of audience.* The general characteristics, such as the demographics of readers, viewers, or listeners of a particular outlet can indicate which information to emphasize or deemphasize and the way to phrase the information. For example, if a media coordinator knows that thirty percent of a readership earns $12,000 annually, the news release could stress the financial need for these persons to vote for the cost containment initiative on an upcoming ballot.
7. *Comprehension level.* Most media outlets gear their material to a specific reading or listening level. Few newspapers write to a readership's maximum potential reading abilities. Rather, they aim for an *average* comfortable level. Hence, knowing the reading or listening level an outlet uses can guide writers of news releases. For example, the writing of many newspapers, perhaps a majority, ranks at the sixth- to eighth-grade level. The *New York Times* ranks at about eleventh-grade reading level. In gen-

eral, the fewer syllables to a word and words to a sentence, the lower the level. A news release that doesn't need recasting to the desired reading level may have greater appeal for a harassed news editor.

8. *Legislative and Congressional districts.* Note what districts the outlet covers. There is little sense in sending a news release to an outlet that isn't interested. For example, endorsement of a candidate in Congressional District 2 or clarification of an issue important to legislative district 13 is useless to an outlet that is not read or viewed in those districts. The news release becomes merely another time waster to an editor or reporter, who may be less inclined to read closely the next release from your organization.

9. *Contacts.* (a) Name, title, and department of the person who is most likely to provide coverage or information; (b) name, title, and department of a backup contact in case the primary contact is vacationing, ill, or otherwise unavailable.

Inquiries to local outlets will yield the names of city editors, healthcare reporters, public service directors, news editors, and editorial page editors or writers. Names for outlets elsewhere are available in the following directories:

Editor and Publisher International Yearbook. Covers both daily and weekly newspapers.
Encyclopedia of Associations, 18th ed.
Ayer's Dictionary of Newspapers and Periodicals.
Bacon's Publicity Checker. Includes major magazines and newspapers.
Gebbie Press House Magazine Directory.
The Broadcasters Yearbook. Covers both radio and television.
Ulrich's International Periodicals Directory.

These references are frequently available in local libraries or local media outlets.

Another source could be the press secretary in the governor's office.

This person usually has a list of regional and local outlets as well as political correspondents for outlets outside the capital. A written request might elicit a copy of this list.

10. *Best time to be in touch.* Indicate the hours during which the person will most likely be available. Mornings are often better for radio and television; afternoons for newspapers. However, your first telephone call should inquire about the hours precisely.
11. *Deadlines.* List deadlines for both copy and photos.
12. *Photo requirements.* Note any requirements differing from or in addition to the standard procedures described on pages 231-232.

For all of this information, a 5-by-8-inch file card works best. This larger size will also allow room for any other pertinent information particular to an outlet.

The card might look like Figure 11.1.

outlet	telephone
address	
Legislative district	Congressional district
contact	2nd contact
best time	best time
scheduled airing/publication	circulation
audience	
comprehension	
deadlines	
photo requirements	

Figure 11.1. *File card*

Release Record. A second kind of file is the record of all releases to the media. The record should list in chronological order every release sent. A looseleaf binder works well for this kind of record. The record should have columns for the release number, date sent, subject, outlet, photos, page or program, and time and date. Place copies of all releases at the back of the binder in chronological order. Be certain to number them to correspond with the numbers on the release record.

A periodic tally of the number of releases each outlet runs will provide useful information for the times when selective focus is imperative. Also, a pattern might become clear: certain outlets might tend to run certain subjects.

Monitoring. A third file consists of articles and summaries of radio and television news reports of interest to your organization, including runs of your releases. A looseleaf binder is best so that the information is removable for photocopying. If any item has prompted a release or correction from your organization, note the numbers from the release record for cross-reference.

Ordering this record according to outlet will provide fast access to the material an outlet has run or to articles a reporter has written. Knowledge of the stories run, their emphasis, and their dates can provide a basis for developing follow-up or related stories. It will also foster a cooperative relationship with the news editors and reporters involved: They will not need to recap and will appreciate your knowledge and interest.

Since monitoring can, in some geographic areas, become a full-time job, assigning people to monitor specific outlets will ensure that little of import escapes notice. It will also lessen the burden and reduce burnout. Monitors should:

1. clip the entire article, including continuation to other pages ("jump")
2. mount articles on 8½-by-11-inch paper (rubber cement works well)
3. identify, in the upper right-hand corner, the outlet, date, and page and column numbers or program and time
4. summarize broadcasted information on 8½-by-11-inch paper

5. send the clipping or summary to the media coordinator, who will distribute photocopies to interested persons and file the article

Media Inquiries. A fourth file should record on cards any inquiries from an outlet. The card should contain the following data: outlet, name, title and department of caller, telephone, date received, date of response, response given, and sources used for verification of response.

Networking with media

Establishing a cooperative relationship with representatives of the media, the identified contacts in particular, is essential. The key idea is cooperation — a joint effort. As with negotiation, you must consider those factors that help the contact as well as your organization. In other words, mere expectation of news coverage for releases and events because they are important to your healthcare organization is insufficient. A contact is not a mere receptacle for news. Rather, a contact is a professional who is building or enhancing a career. Consequently, attention to formats, deadlines, commitments, conciseness, and completeness of information expresses your value not only of the news but also of a contact's time, needs, and professionalism.

To enhance the cooperativeness of the relationship, consider networking — sharing ideas, information, and resources. Your contacts will generally appreciate receiving related and background information, ideas for development of stories, names of persons and articles that can provide further information. Because these media people generally cover subjects other than the health profession, such sharing can include those other subjects as well, for example, passing along information that relates to a story the person has written. The reciprocity that such sharing often develops may result in your contacts' sharing information about breaking stories in the health professions as well as endeavoring to run your releases, to cover your events, and to suggest angles that would increase their newsworthiness.

Other ways of enhancing cooperativeness are compliments and constructive correction. When a reporter writes a good story about issues or events of particular interest to your healthcare profession, call the reporter to say so. Then write a letter to the editor or producer to compliment the paper or station for employing a reporter who does such fine work. Conversely, when a reporter writes a poor story or makes an error, recognize that the cause is usually insufficient information. Call the reporter. Patiently and pleasantly provide the background, related, or correct information that would have improved the story. Include the sources of such information. Going over the reporter's head to the editor or producer is a slur on the reporter's professionalism and can lessen the reporter's future cooperativeness.

To establish or maintain a cooperative relationship, face-to-face communication can be helpful. An informal setting is usually most productive because it excludes the distractions and demands of an office setting. Inviting a reporter for lunch is acceptable. It can provide an opportunity to get acquainted, to discuss a recent or forthcoming story, to supply background information that could provide a context for future stories, and to share information, ideas, and resources. Recognize, however, that journalistic ethics may require reporters to pay their own way.

Usually, however, media people are too busy for a leisurely lunch. If the offer is refused, make an appointment for an office visit or, failing that, a convenient time for a 15 or 20 minute telephone conversation. Have the information or questions handy in case the contact says, "Now is fine." Although face-to-face communication is more personal, media people usually prefer the telephone because it uses less of their time. After any conversation, confirm the details in a brief note and thank the person for the time. If this conversation is a get-acquainted talk, express interest in working with the person in the future.

Remember, media people are constantly working against deadlines. When you phone, (1) have all your points, facts, sources, and questions at hand; (2) be concise in presenting information; and (3) be appreciative. Justified phone calls focus on getting acquainted, on discussing a recent, pending, or potential issue or story, and on offering or requesting information.

Preparation for interviews, news conferences, and panel discussions

Media coordinators should prepare themselves and others for the protocols, questioning, and responses that comprise an interview, news conference, or panel discussion.

Protocols. News conferences are formal events. Media coordinators should identify themselves or other spokesperson(s) by name, title, and affiliation and identify the general subject of the conference. The speaker(s) will read a prepared statement(s). The media coordinator or final speaker will ask for questions at the conclusion of the prepared statements. To facilitate constructive questioning and reporting, all media people should, on arrival, receive a media kit (See page 232).

Interviews are less formal. Provide the interviewer with biographical sketches of the person(s) being interviewed. A list of pertinent questions is also appropriate. At the very least, the list can be a checklist for the interviewer. At most, it can provide a framework for the entire interview. However, interviewers usually have their own lists. If they have interviewed others beforehand, they may have statements for which they want a clarification or a reaction. If the interview is taped, there will be sufficient time off-mike or off-camera to discuss the next series of questions or to urge a particular question. If the interview is live, the interviewer may simply pick up on a sentence or phrase and ask for clarification, elaboration, or the like.

An alert interviewee will ask the interviewer what type of space or time the interview will fill. If the interview is slated for radio or television news, ask whether the interviewer wants a 5, 10, or 20 second answer. For television those times would require about 10, 20 and 40 words, respectively. For radio, one would speak a little faster. Obviously, then a crisp, pithy answer with a beginning, middle, and end is essential. For example: "The legislation, if passed into law [beginning], will increase the consumers' cost of health care [middle] because the health care professionals' operating costs will rise [end]." Do not exploit the question to push your viewpoint. If you think the interview is missing the point, state the point. For example: "The main point, however, is that the legislation, if passed into law, will increase the consumers' cost of health care because the health care professionals' operating expenses will rise."

Panel discussions have a general subject and, usually, specified aspects of the subject. The purpose is to provide the audience with a general understanding of issues, problems, and viewpoints involved. Hence, a panel discussion about cost containment will often include a hospital administrator, a legislator from the health and welfare committee, a consumer advocate, and other persons involved with health care. A moderator will direct questions, summarize, interrupt, and generally keep the discussion moving.

Short, direct responses or summaries of your view or position will lessen the chances of your being interrupted. Interjecting a remark at the end of a panelist's comments is sometimes appropriate. However, the best guide is to watch or listen to the program beforehand to get the pace and the style. If the discussion is a community project, be cautious in the beginning. Sense the flow and the moderator's style. Above all, remain calm and reasoned in your speech. If necessary, just repeat your points. Remember, the purpose of panel discussions is to present views, not to win arguments.

Whether you are responding to questions at a news conference, for an interview, or in a panel discussion, here are some useful guidelines.

1. Do your homework. Have the answers to as many questions as you and your colleagues can think of. Put statistics and specific facts on note cards. Memorize them if you are being televised.

2. Know your questioner. Know for whom the person writes and the type of article or program the person writes. For an interview, read, watch, or listen to a few of the person's stories or programs. Remember, the questioner must interpret and present information in a manner that interests a particular audience.

3. Role play. Training sessions for people who will be or might be speaking to media people ensure relaxed, friendly responses. Practice interviewing, questioning, and panel discussions to familiarize the people with formats and styles as well as to provide practice in answering questions clearly, concisely, and cohesively.

4. Be friendly and responsive to any directions. The questioner's impression of you can guide the questioning or story.

5. Give direct answers to direct questions. If you don't know, say so, but give a source who can supply the answer. "No comment" is a hostile response; "I'm not ready to comment at this time" is an acceptable response. Be prepared, of course, to say why not (you haven't studied the latest report, the data are not yet complete, and so on).

6. Nothing is off the record. You may state, however, that your remarks are "not for attribution." Most media people will

honor this request, and you will become the well-known "reliable source."

7. No question is too basic. Most of the questioner's audience need considerable basic information to become informed.

8. Summarize. Practice summarizing your responses to questions. There usually is not enough time or space for the whole story, and there are deadlines.

9. Stop when you have answered the question. Don't elaborate unless the next question is "Could you clarify that?" Even then, clarify briefly.

10. Speak softly into microphones. In response, the sound crew will usually turn up their microphones. Your voice will sound more intimate, and the effect will bring you closer to the listener's ear and make you seem more important in the listener's imagination.

11. Conclude by thanking the interviewer for his or her time and interest.

News Releases

News releases must inform. They must give facts. The information must have current value to the audience of the outlet. Be selective. Swamping a news editor with releases wastes the editor's time and creates an unfavorable impression. Here are some guidelines.

1. Use 8½-by-11-inch standard, white paper. Use no onionskin (it tears) and no erasable paper (it smears).

2. Type the release on one side of the paper.

3. Put at the top left of page 1:
   - name of person who will answer questions
   - name of organization
   - address
   - day and night telephone numbers for the above named person

4. Put at top right of page 1 the release date and time. Whenever possible use "For immediate release." A specific date should

read, for example, "Release after 2:00 pm, Wednesday, August 22, 1984." "Hold" releases should be used sparingly because they require additional handling and can inadvertently cause complications.

5. Place a headline (summary of contents in *few* words), in all CAPS, ⅓ of the way down the page. The news editor will need the blank space for instructions. The CAPS will call attention to the point you are making.

6. Use 1½ inch margins.

7. Double space.

8. Indent each paragraph at least five spaces.

9. End each page with a complete sentence and a complete paragraph.

10. In the upper right corner, number each page following the first page. In the upper left corner, type the first two or three words of the headline. Type "MORE" at the bottom of all pages except the last page.

11. Type ### or the symbol -30- under the final paragraph. Type "With Art" underneath the symbol if photos or illustrations are included.

12. If an outlet has a style sheet for capitalizing, punctuating, abbreviating, and so on, follow it faithfully. If not, follow the instructions given in a current desk dictionary. Use the dictionary, also, to check spelling.

13. Avoid breaking names of persons, organizations, or places between lines, for example, John-(son), Org-(anization), Wash-(ington).

14. In the first paragraph (the lead), answer the questions *what, who, where, when, why,* and *how.* This paragraph should not exceed eight typed lines.

15. Releases should be no more than two pages, as a general rule.

16. Hand carry news releases to the major outlets. Mail them to other outlets, being certain to mark them to the attention of the contact persons. Double check the media file for deadlines. The release must be received well in advance of such deadlines.

For radio and television, use the above guidelines, modified by the following considerations.

1. Be *very* concise. Frequently the lead paragraph (number 14 above) is sufficient.
2. Use a conversational style. Include phonetic spellings in parentheses after unusual names or terms.
3. Type the release entirely in capital letters.
4. Triple space.
5. Attach a copy of the release sent to the print media. This additional information might be useful to the news editor.

Photographs

With sufficient advance notice a newspaper might send a photographer to cover an event. If so, the media coordinator or a designated person should be on hand to answer questions and provide names and titles of the persons photographed. You may want to hire a photographer if the newspaper can't send one. Get suggestions from the contact person.

Use the following guidelines to ensure usable photographs:

1. Photos showing people interacting have more interest.
2. Newspapers need glossy, black and white photos having sharp contrast.
3. Television outlets prefer color slides, which can be made inexpensively. Otherwise, send a matte or dull-surfaced photo because glossies reflect studio lights.
4. Do not write on the back of the photo.
5. Type the caption on white paper, and attach it by tape to the back of the photo.
   a. Identify the occasion for the photo.
   b. Give full names and initials of all persons, moving from left to right. Include titles only for outstanding guests or a visiting officer of the national organization, or the like;
   c. Fold paper over front of photo;

6. For mailing, place the photo between cardboard, the image facing the back of the envelope. Mark the envelope "Photographs —
Do Not Bend."
7. Retain a copy of each photo for the files.

Media Kits

For any media-covered event, a packet of information and copies of speeches will provide useful facts for a reporter's story. Depending on what the event is, the following items might be useful.

1. news release
2. copies of any speeches given
3. biographical sketches of speakers
4. captioned photos of speakers
5. copies of important statements made by persons not present (senator, mayor, hospital board member)
6. background information; for example, if an issue is licensing, a summary of the issue and the organization's reasons for its stance
7. visual data — charts, tables, statistics, diagrams, copy of research or polls pertinent to the story
8. name and telephone numbers (day and night) of the person whom reporters may call for further information
9. if the covered event announces endorsement of a candidate, include:
   a. biographical sketch of the endorsee
   b. captioned photo of the endorsee
   c. statement from endorsee responding to the endorsement

Media Contacts

To establish effective contacts in the various media, you need to know who does what for each outlet. Then you can select the appropriate media people for your purposes.

For newspapers, the key people are city editors, health writers, editors of editorial pages, writers for editorial pages, and any reporters who might frequently cover healthcare news. A city editor directs the day-to-day news stories and gives assignments to reporters. Consequently, the city editor usually decides which stories get written. A health writer covers all aspects of health care. If a paper has a health writer (many small papers do not), this person should be a top-priority contact. Reporters who frequently cover news about health care would be good contacts, also. The editor of the editorial pages makes the policy about the opinions expressed by the newspaper. Editorial writers cover any topic of current public interest or importance to the community. Their opinions reflect editorial policy. Editorial writers can be valuable contacts because they have the time to develop topics and the space to discuss issues.

In radio and television, the news editor controls the assignment of stories. Public service directors ensure that subjects of community interest and public welfare receive attention. They can arrange special interviews and programs.

Other Kinds of Media Exposure

In addition to news releases, news conferences, interviews, panels, and the day-to-day contact, there are other means of exposure that are sometimes overlooked.

Many areas have weekly or twice-monthly shopper's guides delivered free to residents. These guides sometimes report news or carry features. Or the guides may have a small newspaper accompanying them. In some areas, these guides can be good outlets for news, reports of forthcoming events, and so on.

The electronic media have several kinds of spots worth investigating. Some stations have editorial spots. An owner or manager of a station will deliver an editorial statement about a matter of community concern. Sometimes stations select letters from viewers for airing. Personality announcements are another means of exposure. Some disc jockeys, directors of feature programs, meteorologists, and the like, regularly announce upcoming events. Many stations also make brief announcements throughout the day. Some stations regularly schedule these spots, but others plug them in as fillers when they inadvertently have empty air time. Finally, local TV news broadcasts also might have feature spots toward the end of the program. These short features, 5 minutes at most, might be photographic essays or interviews concerning a matter of community interest or public welfare. They might also report an event that is occurring or forthcoming. The Arizona visiting nurses annually receive coverage for their 3 day book sale. At the same time, TV reporters describe the many services that the visiting nurses perform and in general provide them with a visibility that lingers throughout the year.

Talk shows are another means of reaching an audience. Producers usually book the guests far in advance. Call the stations for information about their procedures for selection if you have information of particular interest or importance to the community.

For all of these spots, inquiries to the station will elicit criteria for selection and requirements for submission of material. If a particular on-air personality is involved, talk to that person.

Summary

The opportunities for communication with media people and exposure in the print and electronic media are many. How much you do depends on your need. Establishing over time the procedures for keeping track of media reporting and features, establishing contacts in the media, and practicing skills necessary for contact or on-air air exposure will provide you with a solid foundation when you need it. Being knowledgeable about the media itself, the particular outlets, and your particular contacts will help you to establish expert power for yourself and your healthcare profession.

Suggestions for Additional Reading

American Nurses Association. *Handbook for political media.* Washington, DC: Author, n.d.

Archer, S., and Goehner, P. *Nurses: A political force.* Monterey, CA: Wadsworth, Inc., 1982.

Brown, C. J., Brown, T. R., and Rivers, W. L. *The media and the people.* Huntington, NY: Robert E. Krieger Publishing Co., 1978.

Fox, D. *The politics of city, state, and bureaucracy.* Pacific Palisades, CA: Goodyear Publishing Co., 1974.

Francois, W. *Mass media law and regulation.* Columbus, OH: Grid, Inc., 1978.

Graber, D. A. *Mass media and American politics.* Washington, DC: Congressional Quarterly, Inc., 1980.

Lemert, J. B. *Does mass communication change public opinion after all?* Chicago: Nelson-Hall, 1981.

N-CAP. Time for nurses to make a difference through politics. Washington, DC: N-CAP, 1981.

Pember, D. *Mass media law.* Dubuque, IA: William C. Brown, 1981.

Appendix A: National and State Political Resources

This appendix gives a brief listing of several resources for information concerning federal and state legislatures and agencies.

Federal Resources

Federal records offices

Copies of federal campaign finance reports may be reviewed and copied at the following locations:

All Reports
Public Records Division
Federal Election Commission
1325 K Street, N.W.
Washington, DC 20463
202/523-4181
$.05–.10/pg.

Note: These reports are made available for public review and copying, provided that any information copied from these reports shall not be sold or used by any person for the purpose of soliciting contributions or for any commercial purpose, other than using the name and address of any political committee to solicit contributions from such committees. 2 U.S.C. 438(a)(4).

U.S. Senate Reports
Office of Public Records
Office of the Secretary of the Senate
119 D Street, N.E.
Washington, DC 20510
202/224-0322
$.10/pg.

U.S. House of Representatives Reports
Office of Records and Registration
Office of the Clerk of the House
Longworth House Office Bldg., Rm. 1036
Washington, DC 20515
202/225-1300
$.10/pg.

Party headquarters

Association of State Democratic Chairs
1625 Massachusetts Avenue, N.W.
Washington, DC 20036
202/797-6549

Dwight D. Eisenhower Republican Center
310 First Street Southeast
Washington, DC 20003
202/863-8500

Federal toll-free and commercial numbers

These federal agencies could provide information that is pertinent to current issues and to concerns of members of networks and coalitions.

Banking
Federal Deposit Insurance Corporation
202/389-4353 (Washington, DC)
1/800/424-5488 (Elsewhere)
Hours: 9:00–5:00, Mon.–Fri.

Receives complaints and provides information on the consumer banking laws.

Federal Home Loan Bank Board
202/377-6988 (Washington, DC)
1/800/424-5405 (Elsewhere)
Hours: 24 hour recording

Provides information on federal adjustable mortgage rates.

Child Abuse
Parents Anonymous
1/800/352-0386 (California)
1/800/421-0353 (Elsewhere)

Counseling and advice for parents and others concerned about child abuse.

Cooperative Extension Service. The Cooperative Extension Service is a three-way partnership involving the U.S. Department of Agriculture, the state land-grant universities, and county governments. The Extension staff provides information and education programs for children and adults on food, nutrition, gardening, money management and a variety of other subjects. To find your local listing, consult the telephone directory under your state's land-grant university or your county government.

Education
Student Information Center
Department of Education
301/984-4070 (Maryland and Elsewhere)
Hours: 9:00–5:30 Mon.–Fri. (Eastern Time)

Provides information on postsecondary financial aid opportunities.

Energy
Conservation and Renewable Energy
Inquiry Referral Service
1/800/462-4983 (Pennsylvania)
1/800/233-3071 (Alaska and Hawaii)

1/800/523-2929 (Elsewhere)
Hours: 9:00–5:00 Mon.–Fri. (Eastern Time)

Provides nontechnical information on solar, wind, and other energy heating and cooling technologies, energy conservation and alcohol fuels.

National Ride-Sharing Information Center
Federal Highway Administration
Department of Transportation
202/426-0210
(800 number discontinued)

Provides information on ride sharing, but not on rider-matching service.

Environment
Hazardous Waste
Environmental Protection Agency
202/382-3000 (Washington, DC)
1/800/424-9346 (Elsewhere)
Hours: 8:30–4:30, Mon.–Fri. (Eastern Time)

Provides information on hazardous waste.

Pesticide Hotline
Environmental Protection Agency
1/800/292-7664 (Texas)
1/800/531-7790 (Elsewhere)
Hours: 9:00–5:00 Mon.–Fri. (Central Time)

Provides information on pesticides.

Handicapped
Library of Congress
202/287-5100 (Washington, DC)
1/800/424-9100 (Elsewhere)
Hours: 8:00–4:30 Mon.–Fri.
Answering service after hours.

Provides information on programs and books for the blind and physically handicapped.

Health Care
Low Income Assistance
Hill-Burton Hospitals
Department of Health and Human Services
1/800/492-0359 (Maryland)
1/800/638-0742 (Elsewhere)
Hours: 9:00–5:00 Mon.–Fri.

Receives inquiries about Hill-Burton hospitals (hospitals required by law to provide free or reduced charges to those who qualify because of low income).

Cancer Information Service
National Cancer Institute
National Institutes of Health
Department of Health and Human Services
202/636-5700 (Washington, DC)
1/800/4 CANCER (Maryland)
1/800/794-7982 (N.Y. City)
1/800/638-6070 (Alaska)
1/800/524-1234 (Hawaii)
Hours: 9:00–5:00 Mon.–Fri.

Provides information on cancer treatment and ongoing research; fills requests for pamphlets and other literature on cancer.

National Health Information Clearinghouse
Department of Health and Human Services
703/522-2590 (Washington, DC, Virginia, Alaska, and Hawaii)
Residents of Virginia, Alaska, and Hawaii can call collect.
1/800/336-4797 (Elsewhere)
Hours: 8:30–5:00 Mon.–Fri.
Answering service after hours.

Provides referrals to sources of information on health-related issues.

Highway Safety
National Highway Traffic Safety Administration
Department of Transportation
202/426-0123 (Washington, DC)
1/800/424-9393 (Elsewhere)
Hours: 7:45–4:15 Mon.–Fri.
Answering service after hours.

Provides information on motor vehicle safety recalls; handles complaints on safety-related defects; and receives reports of vehicle safety problems.

Housing
Fair Housing and Equal Opportunity
Department of Housing and Urban Development
202/426-3500 (Washington, DC)
1/800/424-8590 (Elsewhere)
Hours: 8:45–5:15 Mon.–Fri.
Answering service after hours.

Insurance
Federal Crime Insurance
Department of Housing and Urban Development
202/652-2637 (Washington, DC and Maryland. Will accept toll
    calls from MD)
1/800/638-8780 (Elsewhere)
Hours: 9:00–5:00 Mon.–Fri.
Answering service after hours.

Provides information on federal crime insurance for both homes and businesses.

Federal Flood Insurance
Federal Emergency Management Administration
301/731-5300 (Washington, DC Area)
1/800/492-6605 (Maryland)

1/800/638-6831 (Alaska, Hawaii, Puerto Rico, Virgin Islands)
1/800/638-6620 (Elsewhere)
Hours: 8:00–4:30 Mon.–Fri.

Provides information on community participation in the flood program (emergency or regular). If the community does not have a program, it is not eligible for government subsidized insurance relief. Complaints are referred to the proper office within the agency.

Product Safety
Consumer Product Safety Commission
1/800/638-2772 (Maryland, Alaska, Hawaii, Puerto Rico, Virgin
  Islands, Elsewhere)
Teletype available for the deaf.
1/800/492-8104 (Maryland)
1/800/638-8270 (Elsewhere)
Hours: 8:30–5:00 Mon.–Fri.
Answering service after hours.

Provides information on the comparative safety consumer products. Receives reports of product-related deaths, illnesses, and injuries.

Social Security. The Social Security Administration has a system of regional offices that can be called without long-distance expense to the consumer. To find out your local 800 number or tie line number, consult your telephone directory or local directory assistance operator.

Taxes. The Internal Revenue Service has regional and district offices that can be called without long-distance expense. To find out your local number, consult your telephone directory or local directory assistance operator.

Federal information centers

For information and help with your questions about the federal government, use the following list to find the nearest Federal Information Center (part of the U.S. General Services Administration).

Please call the listing closest to you for a free call or minimum long-distance charge.

Telephone Numbers

Alabama
    Birmingham 205/322-8591
    Mobile 205/438-1421

Alaska
    Anchorage 907/271-3650

Arizona
    Phoenix 602/261-3313

Arkansas
    Little Rock 501/378-6177

California
    Los Angeles 213/688-3800
    Sacramento 916/440-3344
    San Diego 619/293-6030
    San Francisco 415/556-6600
    Santa Ana 714/836-2386

Colorado
    Colorado Springs 303/471-9491
    Denver 303/236-7181
    Pueblo 303/544-9523

Connecticut
    Hartford 203/527-2617
    New Haven 203/624-4720

Florida
    Ft. Lauderdale 305/522-8531
    Jacksonville 904/354-4756
    Miami 305/350-4155

Orlando 305/422-1800
St. Petersburg 813/893-3495
Tampa 813/229-7911
West Palm Beach 305/833-7566

Georgia
Atlanta 404/221-6891

Hawaii
Honolulu 808/546-8620

Illinois
Chicago 312/353-4242

Indiana
Gary 219/883-4110
Indianapolis 317/269-7373

Iowa
From all points in Iowa
1/800/532-1556

Kansas
From all points in Kansas
1/800/432-2934

Kentucky
Louisville 502/582-6261

Louisiana
New Orleans 504/589-6696

Maryland
Baltimore 301/962-4980

Massachusetts
Boston 617/223-7121

Michigan
Detroit 313/226-7016
Grand Rapids 616/451-2628

Minnesota
Minneapolis 612/349-5333

Missouri
St. Louis 314/425-4106
From elsewhere in Missouri
1/800/392-7711

Nebraska
Omaha 402/221-3353
From elsewhere in Nebraska
1/800/642-8383

New Jersey
Newark 201/645-3600
Trenton 609/396-4400

New Mexico
Albuquerque 505/766-3091

New York
Albany 518/463-4421
Buffalo 716/846-4010
New York 212/264-4464
Rochester 716/546-5075
Syracuse 315/476-8545

North Carolina
Charlotte 704/376-3600

Ohio
Akron 216/375-5638
Cincinnati 513/684-2801

Cleveland 216/522-4040
Columbus 614/221-1014
Dayton 513/223-7377
Toledo 419/241-3223

Oklahoma
Oklahoma City 405/231-4868
Tulsa 918/584-4193

Oregon
Portland 503/221-2222

Pennsylvania
Philadelphia 215/597-7042
Pittsburgh 412/644-3456

Rhode Island
Providence 401/331-5565

Tennessee
Chattanooga 615/265-8231
Memphis 901/521-3285
Nashville 615/242-5056

Texas
Austin 512/472-5494
Dallas 214/767-8585
Fort Worth 817/334-3624
Houston 713/229-2552
San Antonio 512/224-4471

Utah
Salt Lake City 801/524-5353

Virginia
Norfolk 804/441-3101
Richmond 804/643-4928
Roanoke 703/982-8591

Washington
  Seattle 206/442-0570
  Tacoma 206/383-5230

Wisconsin
  Milwaukee 414/271-2273

State Resources

This listing contains the following resources:

- the toll-free state consumer telephone numbers of the thirty-two states having this office
- Democratic and Republican Party Headquarters address and telephone
- secretary of state address and telephone
  From this office you can obtain information about the operation of your state. You can also obtain the legislative information telephone number at your state legislature. (In Alaska and Hawaii, the office of the lieutenant governor handles the duties of secretary of state.)
- State election office address and telephone
  This office provides information concerning state election laws and procedures, including PACs, campaign funds and finance reports, petitions, district and precincts, and so on. If an office is not separately listed, call the secretary of state.

Alabama
Alabama (Montgomery)
Hours: 8:00–5:00
1/800/392-5658
In-state only. Advice given over the phone. Complaints must be submitted in writing for action.

Alabama Democratic Headquarters
306 Jefferson Federal Building

Birmingham, AL 35203
205/252-4143

The Alabama Republican Executive Committee
Post Office Box 31046, Birmingham 35222
205/324-1984

Office of the Secretary of State
State Capitol
Montgomery, AL 36130
205/832-3570

Secretary of State
Elections Division
State Capitol
Montgomery, AL 36130
205/832-3570

Alaska
Alaska Democratic Headquarters
P.O. Box 10-4199
Anchorage, AK 99510
907/563-6480

Republican Party of Alaska
515 "D" Street — Suite 203
Anchorage, AK 99501
907/276-4467

Office of the Lt. Governor
State Capitol
3rd floor
Pouch AA
Juneau, AK 99811
907/465-3520

Arizona

Arizona (Phoenix)
Hours: 8:00–5:00
1/800/352-8431
In-state only. Handles complaints concerning possible fraud.

Arizona Democratic Headquarters
1001 N. Central, #107
Phoenix, AZ 85004
602/257-9136

Arizona Republican State Committee
40 East Thomas, Suite 100
Phoenix, AZ 85012
602/248-8484

Secretary of State
Department of State
State Capitol, W. Wing
Phoenix, AZ 85007
602/255-4285

Office of the Secretary of State
1700 W. Washington, West Wing
Suite 700
Phoenix, AZ 85007
602/255-4285

Arkansas

Arkansas (Little Rock)
Hours: 8:00–5:00
1/800/482-8982
In-state only. Handles complaints concerning possible fraud or false
advertising and will answer general inquiries.

Arkansas Democratic Headquarters
1300 West Capitol

Little Rock, AR 72201
501/374-2361

Republican Party of Arkansas
Twin City Bank Bldg.
1 River Front Place
Suite 620
North Little Rock, AR 72114
501/372-7301

Office of the Secretary of State
256 State Capitol Bldg.
Little Rock, AR 72201
501/371-1010

Election Division, Room 026
Office of the Secretary of State
256 State Capitol Building
Little Rock, AR 72201
501/371-5070

California
California (Sacramento)
Hours: 8:00–5:00
1/800/952-5210
In-state only. Handles complaints concerning auto repair jobs.
1/800/952-5670
In-state only. Information regarding solar energy uses/taxes.
1/800/822-6228
General energy information.
Hours: 9:00–12:00; 1:00–4:00
1/800/952-5225
In-state only. Takes general opinions.

California Democratic Headquarters
9911 West Pico, #301
Los Angeles, CA 90035
213/201-0123

California Republican Party
1228 N Street, Sacramento 95814
916/443-0967
4002 Burbank Boulevard
Burbank, CA 91505
213/841-5252

Office of the Secretary of State
1230 J Street
Sacramento, CA 95814

Political Reform Division
Office of the Secretary of State
1230 J Street
P.O. Box 1467
Sacramento, CA 95807
916/322-4880

Colorado
Colorado Democratic Headquarters
1835 Race Street
Denver, CO 80206
303/320-1000
Executive Director: Sherrie Wolff

Republican State Central
Committee of Colorado
1275 Tremont Place
Denver, CO 80204
303/893-1776

Office of the Secretary of State
Social Services Bldg., 2nd Fl.
1575 Sherman Street
Denver, CO 80203
303/866-5000

Elections Division
Office of the Secretary of State
1575 Sherman Street, Rm. 211
Denver, CO 80203
303/862-2041

Connecticut
Connecticut (Hartford)
Hours: 8:30–4:30
1/800/842-2649
In-state only. Handles all types of complaints and inquiries.

Connecticut Democratic Headquarters
634 Asylum Avenue
Hartford, CT 06105
203/278-6080

Connecticut Republicans
1 High Street
Hartford, CT 06103
203/249-9661

The Hon. Julia H. Tashjian
Office of the Secretary of State
State Capitol, Room 106
Hartford, CT 06115
203/566-4135

Administrative/Legislative Division
Office of the Secretary of State
30 Trinity Street
Hartford, CT 06115
203/566-3059

Delaware
Delaware Democratic Headquarters
Radisson Hotel, Suite 8

Wilmington, DE 19807
302/552-1984

Delaware Republican State Committee
2008 Pennsylvania Avenue, Suite 208
Wilmington, DE 19806
302/652-3132

Office of the Secretary of State
Townsend Bldg.
Dover, DE 19901
302/736-4111

District of Columbia
D.C. Democratic Headquarters
1110 Vermont Avenue, N.W. #840
Washington, DC 20005
202/347-5670

District of Columbia Republican Committee
1700 K Street, N.W., Suite 1102
Washington, DC 20006

Florida
Florida (Tallahassee)
Hours: 7:45-4:30 (recording after hours)
1/800/342-2176
In-state only. Handles most types of complaints and inquiries.

Florida Democratic Headquarters
P.O. Box 1758
Tallahassee, FL 32302
904/222-3411

Republican State Executive Committee of Florida
P.O. Box 311
Tallahassee, FL 32302 (103 Call Street)
904/222-7290

Department of State
The Capitol
Tallahassee, FL 33201
904/488-7690

Georgia
Georgia (Atlanta)
Hours: 8:00–5:00
1/800/282-5808
In-state only. Handles general complaints and inquiries.

Georgia Democratic Headquarters
901 South Omni International
Atlanta, GA 30303
404/688-1984

Georgia Republican Party
1951 Airport Road, Suite 200
Atlanta, GA 30341
404/458-0293

Office of the Secretary of State
State Capitol
Atlanta, GA 30334
404/656-2881

State Elections Division
Office of the Secretary of State
State Capitol, Rm. 224
Atlanta, GA 30334
404/656-2871

Hawaii
Hawaii Democratic Headquarters
33 S. King Street, Suite 216
Honolulu, HI 96813
1/808/536-2258

Republican Party of Hawaii
1136 Union Mall, Room 203
Honolulu, HI 96813
1/808/526-1755

Office of the Lt. Governor
State Capitol, 5th Fl.
Honolulu, HI 96813
1/808/548-2544

Campaign Spending Commission
State Capitol, Rm. 008
P.O. Box 501
Honolulu, HI 96809
1/808/548-5411

Idaho
Idaho Democratic Headquarters
Box 445
Boise, ID 83701
208/336-1815

Idaho Republican State Central Committee
P.O. Box 2267
Boise, ID 83701
208/343-6405

Office of the Secretary of State
State Capitol, Room 203
Boise, ID 83720
208/334-2300

Elections Division
Office of the Secretary of State
State House, Rm. 205
Boise, ID 83720
208/334-2300

Illinois

Illinois (Chicago)

1/800/252-8980

In-state only. Handles complaints and inquiries on used car ownership, titles, and licenses.

1/800/252-8903

In-state only. Handles complaints and inquiries on public aid fraud.

Illinois Democratic Headquarters

534 S. 2nd Street

Springfield, IL 62701

217/528-3471 or 217/782-3905

Illinois Republican State Central Committee

200 South Second Street

Springfield, IL 62701

217/525-0011

Cook County Office:

127 N. Dearborn St., Rm. 828

Chicago, IL 60602

312/641-6400

Office of the Secretary of State

213 State Capitol

Springfield, IL 62706

217/782-2201

State Board of Elections

1020 S. Spring Street

P.O. Box 4187

Springfield, IL 62708

217/782-4141

Indiana

Indiana (Indianapolis)

Hours: 8:15–4:45

1/800/382-5516

In-state only. Handles general consumer complaints and inquiries.

Indiana Democratic Headquarters
47 E. Washington Street — Lower Level
Indianapolis, IN 46204
317/635-8581

Indiana Republican State Central Committee
150 West Market St., Suite 200
Indianapolis, IN 46204
317/635-7561

Office of the Secretary of State
201 State House
Indianapolis, IN 46204
317/232-6531

Iowa
Iowa Democratic Headquarters
1120 Mulberry Street
Des Moines, IA 50309
515/244-7292

Republican State Central Committee of Iowa
1540 High Street
Des Moines, IA 50309
515/282-8105

Office of the Secretary of State
State House
Des Moines, IA 50319
515/281-5864

Campaign Finance Disclosure Commission
1st Floor, Colony Building
507 10th Street
Des Moines, IA 50309
515/281-4411

Kansas

Kansas (Topeka)
Hours: 8:00–5:00
1/800/432-2310
In-state only. Handles general complaints and inquiries.

Kansas Democratic Headquarters
P.O. Box 1914
Topeka, KS 66601
913/234-0425

Kansas Republican State Committee
Suite 22
501 Jefferson
Topeka, KS 66607
913/234-3416

Office of the Secretary of State
State House, 2nd Floor
Topeka, KS 66612
913/296-2236

Kentucky

Kentucky (Frankfort)
Hours: 8:30–5:00
1/800/432-9527
In-state only. Advice given over the phone. Will send complaint
    forms or refer.

Kentucky Democratic Headquarters
P.O. Box 964
Frankfort, KY 40602
502/695-4828

Republican Party of Kentucky
Capitol Avenue at Third

Frankfort, KY 40601
502/875-5130

Office of the Secretary of State
Capitol Bldg.
Frankfort, KY 40601
502/564-3490

Kentucky Registry of Election Finance
1604 Louisville Road
Frankfort, KY 40601
502/564-2226

Louisiana
Louisiana (Baton Rouge)
Hours: 8:30–5:00
1/800/272-9868
In-state only. Handles general complaints and inquiries.

Louisiana Democratic Headquarters
3080 Teddy Drive, Suite B
Baton Rouge, LA 70809
504/926-3110

The Republican Party of Louisiana
650 North 6th Street
Baton Rouge, LA 70802
504/383-7234

Office of the Secretary of State
State Capitol Building, 14th Floor
P.O. Box 44125 — Capitol Station
Baton Rouge, LA 70804
504/342-5710

Maine
Maine Democratic Headquarters
2 Central Plaza

Augusta, ME 04330
207/622-6233

Maine Republican State Committee
51 Chapel Street
Augusta, ME 04330
207/622-6247

Department of the Secretary of State
State House, Station #101
Augusta, ME 04333
207/289-3501

Election Division
Office of the Secretary of State
State Office Building
Augusta, ME 04333
207/289-3501

Maryland
Maryland Democratic Headquarters
123 W. Read Street
Baltimore, MD 21201
301/539-1500

Republican State Central Committee of Maryland
60 West Street, Suite 201
Annapolis, MD 21401
301/269-0113

Office of the Secretary of State
Executive Department
State House
Annapolis, MD 21404
301/269-3421

State Administration Board of Election Laws
11 Bladen Street

P.O. Box 231
Annapolis, MD 21404
301/269-3711

Massachusetts
Massachusetts (Boston)
Hours: 9:00–5:00
1/800/632-8026
In-state only. Handles energy-related complaints and concerns.
1/800/392-6066
In-state only. Handles public utility complaints and inquiries.

Massachusetts Democratic Headquarters
11 Beacon Street, Suite 317
Boston, MA 02108
617/367-4760

Massachusetts Republican State Committee
73 Tremont Street, Room 927
Boston, MA 02108
617/523-7535

Office of the Secretary of Commonwealth
State House, Room 337
Boston, MA 01233
617/727-2800

Division of Public Records
Office of the Secretary of State
1701–1703 McCormack Bldg.
One Ashburton Place
Boston, MA 01208
617/727-2832

Michigan
Michigan (Lansing)
Hours: 8:30–5:00

1/800/292-4204 (Bureau of Automotive Regulation)
In-state only. Handles auto complaints.
1/800/292-9555 (Public Service Commission)
In-state only. Handles utility-related complaints.

Michigan Democratic Headquarters
606 Townsend
Lansing, MI 48933
517/371-5410

Michigan Republican Committee
223 North Walnut Street
Lansing, MI 48933
517/487-5413

Office of the Secretary of State
Department of State
Treasury Bldg., 1st Fl.
Lansing, MI 48918
517/373-2510

Elections Division
Office of the Secretary of State
208 N. Capitol Avenue
P.O. Box 20126
Lansing, MI 48918
517/373-8558

Minnesota
Minnesota Democratic Headquarters
730 East 38th Street
Minneapolis, MN 55407
612/827-5421

Independent — Republicans of Minnesota
555 Wabasha Street
St. Paul, MN 55102
612/291-1286

Secretary of State
Office of the Secretary of State
180 State Office Bldg.
St. Paul, MN 55155
612/296-2079

Office of the Secretary of State
180 State Office Bldg.
St. Paul, MN 55155
612/296-2805

Mississippi
Mississippi (Jackson)
Hours: 8:00-5:00
1/800/222-7622 (Governor's Hotline)
In-state only. Consumer complaints are referred.

Mississippi Democratic Headquarters
P.O. Box 1583
Jackson, MS 39205
601/969-2913

Mississippi Republican Party
P.O. Box 1178
Jackson, MS 39205
601/948-5191

Office of the Secretary of State
New Capitol, Room 106
P.O. Box 136
Jackson, MS 39205
601/334-6541

Missouri
Missouri (Jefferson City)
Hours: 8:15-4:45

1/800/392-8222
In-state only. Handles complaints involving fraud and misrepresentations in the sale of goods.

Missouri Democratic Headquarters
P.O. Box 719
Jefferson City, MO 65101
314/636-5241

Missouri Republican State Committee
P.O. Box 73
Jefferson City, MO 65101
314/636-3146

Office of the Secretary of State
209 State Capitol
P.O. Box 778
Jefferson City, MO 65102
314/751-2379

Division of Campaign Financing
Office of the Secretary of State
Jefferson City, MO 65101
314/751-3077

Montana
Montana (Helena)
Hours: 8:00–5:00 (answering service after hours)
1/800/332-2272
In-state only. Refers complaints and inquiries to the proper state
    office.

Montana Democratic Headquarters
P.O. Box 802
Helena, MT 59624
406/442-9520

Montana Republican State Central Committee
1425 Helena Avenue
Helena, MT 59601
406/442-6469

Office of the Secretary of State
State Capitol, Room 202
Helena, MT 59620
406/449-2034

Commission on Political Practices
1205 8th Street
Helena, MT 59601
406/449-2942

Nebraska
Nebraska Democratic Headquarters
715 South 14th Street
Lincoln, NE 68508
402/475-4584

Nebraska Republican State Central Committee
421 South 9th Street, Suite 102
Lincoln, NE 68508
402/475-2122

Office of the Secretary of State
State Capitol, Room 2300
Lincoln, NE 68509
402/471-2554

Nevada
Nevada (Carson City)
Hours: 8:00–5:00
1/800/992-0973
In-state only. Operator connects consumer with state agencies. Consumer must know which agency to request.

Nevada Democratic Headquarters
506 Humboldt Street
Reno, NV 89509
702/323-8683

Republican State Central Committee of Nevada
P.O. Box 1888
Carson City, NV 89702
702/885-9115

Office of the Secretary of State
Capitol Bldg.
Carson City, NV 89710
702/885-5203

New Hampshire
New Hampshire (Concord)
Hours: 8:00–4:00
1/800/852-3456 (Governor's Office of Citizens Services)
In-state only. Handles complaints and inquiries concerning energy.
1/800/852-3311 (State Human Resources Division)
Insurance Department Complaint Line
1/800/852-3416
In-state only. Refers complaints and inquiries to the proper state
   office.

New Hampshire Democratic Headquarters
922 Elm Street, #210
Manchester, NH 03101
603/622-9606

New Hampshire Republican State Committee
134 North Main Street
Concord, NH 03301
603/225-9341

Office of the Secretary of State
State House, Room 204

Concord, NH 03301
603/271-3242

New Jersey
New Jersey (Trenton)
Hours: 9:00–5:00 (recording after hours)
1/800/792-8600
In-state only. Refers complaints and inquiries to the proper agency.

New Jersey Democratic Headquarters
Capitol Plaza Hotel — 15th Floor
240 West State Street
Trenton, NJ 08060
609/392-3367

New Jersey Republican State Committee
312 West State Street
Trenton, NJ 08618
609/989-7300

Office of the Secretary of State
Department of State
CN-300
Trenton, NJ 08625
609/292-3790

Election Section
Department of State
107 West State Street
Trenton, NJ 08625
609/292-3790

New Mexico
New Mexico Democratic Headquarters
621 Rio Grande Blvd., N.W.
Albuquerque, NM 87104
505/243-9571

Republican State Central Committee of New Mexico
3701 San Mateo, N.E., — Suite F
Albuquerque, NM 87110
505/265-1984

Office of the Secretary of State
State Capitol, Room 400
Sante Fe, NM 87503
505/827-3601

New York
New York (Albany)
Hours: 7:30–4:30
1/800/342-3736
In-state only. Handles consumer inquiries on all types of insurance coverage.
Hours: 9:00–5:00
1/800/342-3377
In-state only. Refers consumer inquiries on utilities to the proper public service/utility.
Hours: 7:30–4:30
1/800/342-3823
In-state only. Handles complaints concerning auto repairs performed within the last 90 days.
Hours: 9:00–4:00
1/800/342-3722 (recording after hours)
In-state only. Answers inquiries about energy programs, conservation, and regulations.
Hours: 7:30–9:30
1/800/342-3355
Utility emergencies.

New York Democratic Headquarters
60 East 42nd Street
New York, NY 10165
212/986-2955

New York Republican State Committee
315 State Street
Albany, NY 12210
518/462-2601

Office of the Secretary of State
State Department
162 Washington Avenue
Albany, NY 12231
518/474-4750

State Board of Elections Agency
99 Washington Avenue
Albany, NY 12210
518/474-8200

North Carolina
North Carolina (Raleigh)
Hours: 8:00–5:00
1/800/662-7777
In-state only. Receives inquiries about insurance coverage.

North Carolina Democratic Headquarters
P.O. Box 12196
Raleigh, NC 27605
919/821-2777

North Carolina Republican Executive Committee
P.O. Box 12905
Raleigh, NC 27605
919/828-6423

Office of the Secretary of State
State Capitol
Raleigh, NC 27611
919/733-3434

Campaign Reporting Office
State Board of Elections
Raleigh Building, Rm. 809
5 W. Hargett St., P.O. Box 1934
Raleigh, NC 27602
919/733-2186

North Dakota
North Dakota (Bismarck)
Hours: 8:00–5:00
1/800/472-2600
In-state only. Investigates allegations of consumer fraud.
Hours: 8:00–5:00
1/800/472-2600
In-state only. Handles general consumer complaints.

North Dakota Democratic Headquarters
1902 East Divide Avenue
Bismarck, ND 58501
701/255-0460

North Dakota Republican State Committee
P.O. Box 1917
Russel Building Highway 83N
Bismarck, ND 58502
701/255-0030

Office of the Secretary of State
State Capitol, 1st Fl.
Bismarck, ND 58505
701/224-2900

Ohio
Ohio (Columbus)
Hours: 8:00–5:00 (recording after hours)
1/800/282-0515
In-state only. Handles general complaints and inquiries.

Ohio Democratic Headquarters
88 East Broad Street
Suite 1920
Columbus, OH 43215
514/221-6563

Republican State Central and Executive Committee of Ohio
50 West Broad Street
Columbus, OH 43215
614/228-2481

Office of the Secretary of State
State Office Tower, 14th Floor
30 East Broad Street
Columbus, OH 43216
614/466-2585

Oklahoma

Oklahoma (Oklahoma City)
Hours: 8:00–5:00
1/800/522-8555 (Capitol Straight Line)
In-state only. Handles general complaints and inquiries.
1/800/522-8154
Inquiries on public utilities.

Oklahoma Democratic Headquarters
4545 N. Lincoln, Suite 66
Oklahoma City, OK 73105
405/524-1400

Republican State Committee of Oklahoma
123 Northwest 23rd Street
Oklahoma City, OK 73103
405/528-3501

Oregon

Oregon Democratic Headquarters
P.O. Box 1012

Salem, OR 97308
503/370-8200

Oregon Republican State Central Committee
18791 South West Martinazzi
Tualatin, OR 97062
or Post Office Box 848
Tualatin, OR 97062
503/692-0616

Office of the Secretary of State
136 State Capitol
Salem, OR 97310
503/378-4139

Elections Division
Office of the Secretary of State
State Capitol, Rm. 141
Salem, OR 97310
503/378-4144

Pennsylvania
Pennsylvania Democratic Headquarters
510 North 3rd Street
Harrisburg, PA 17101
717/238-9381

Republican State Committee of Pennsylvania
P.O. Box 1624
(112 State Street)
Harrisburg, PA 17105
717/234-4901

Office of the Secretary of State
Department of State
302 North Office Bldg.
Harrisburg, PA 17120
717/787-7630

Bureau of Elections
North Office Building, Rm. 305
Harrisburg, PA 17120
717/787-5280

Rhode Island

Rhode Island Democratic Headquarters
Charles Orm Bldg., Suite 328
10 Orm Street
Providence, RI 02904
401/273-8700

Rhode Island State Central Committee
146 Westminster Street
Providence, RI 02903
401/421-2570

Office of the Secretary of State
State Capitol
Providence, RI 02903
401/277-2357

Elections Division
Office of the Secretary of State
State House, Rm. 16
Providence, RI 02903
401/277-2340

South Carolina

South Carolina (Columbia)
Hours: 8:00–5:00
1/800/922-1594
In-state only. Handles general complaints and inquiries.

South Carolina Democratic Headquarters
711 Whaley Street
Columbia, SC 29201
803/799-7798

The South Carolina Republican Party
P.O. Box 5247
(616 Harden Street)
Columbia, SC 29250
803/799-1610

Office of the Secretary of State
P.O. Box 11350
Columbia, SC 28211
803/758-2744

State Election Commission
2221 Devine Street, Room 105
P.O. Box 5987
Columbia, SC 29250
803/758-2571

South Dakota
South Dakota (Pierre)
Hours: 8:00–5:00
1/800/592-1865
In-state only. Must ask for specific division.

South Dakota Democratic Headquarters
P.O. Box 668
Pierre, SD 57501
605/224-8638

South Dakota Republican State Central Committee
P.O. Box 1099
(221 South Central)
Pierre, SD 57501
605/224-7347

Office of the Secretary of State
Capitol Building, 2nd Fl.
Pierre, SD 57501
605/773-3537

Tennessee

Tennessee (Nashville)
Hours: 8:00–4:30
1/800/342-8385
In-state only. Handles general complaints and inquiries.

Tennessee Democratic Headquarters
205 7th Avenue N.
Nashville, TN 37219
615/244-1336

Tennessee Republican State Executive Committee
3815 Cleghorn Avenue
Nashville, TN 37215
615/383-7890

Office of the Secretary of State
State Capitol
Nashville, TN 37219
615/741-2816

State Library & Archives
403 7th Avenue North, Room 200
Nashville, TN 37219
615/741-2451

Texas

Texas Democratic Headquarters
305 Stokes Building
11th & Guadalupe
Austin, TX 78701
512/478-8746

Republican Party of Texas
1300 Guadalupe, Suite 205
Austin, TX 78701
512/477-9821

Office of the Secretary of State
P.O. Box 12887
Austin, TX 78701
512/475-4434

Elections Division
Office of the Secretary of State
State Capitol, Room 127
Box 12887
Austin, TX 78711
512/475-5619

Utah
Utah Democratic Headquarters
849 East 400 South
Salt Lake City, UT 84102
801/328-0239

Utah Republican State Central Committee
643 East 4th South, Suite A
Salt Lake City, UT 84012
801/533-9777

Office of the Secretary of State
203 State Capitol Building
Salt Lake City, UT 84114
801/533-5115

Vermont
Vermont (Montpelier)
Hours: 8:00–4:30
1/800/642-5149
In-state only. Handles general complaints and inquiries.

Vermont Democratic Headquarters
109 South Winooski Ave.
Suite 207
Burlington, VT 05401
802/864-0431

Vermont Republican State Committee
P.O. Box 70
(100 State Street)
Montpelier, VT 05602
802/223-3411

Office of the Secretary of State
Pavillion Office Building
Montpelier, VT 05602
802/828-2363

Virginia
Virginia (Richmond)
Hours: 8:30–5:00
1/800/552-9963
In-state only. Handles general complaints and inquiries.

Virginia Democratic Headquarters
701 E. Franklin Street, Suite 801
Richmond, VA 23219
804/544-1966

Republican Party of Virginia
115 East Grace Street
Richmond, VA 23219
804/780-0111

Office of the Secretary of the Commonwealth
Ninth St. Office Bldg.
Richmond, VA 23219
804/786-2441

State Board of Elections
101 Ninth Street Office Bldg.
Richmond, VA 23219
804/786-6551

Washington

Washington (Seattle)
Hours: 1:00-5:00
1/800/552-4630
In-state only. Will mail out complaint forms or make referrals.

Washington Democratic Headquarters
P.O. Box 4027
Seattle, WA 98104
206/583-0664

Republican State Committee of Washington
Nine Lake Bellevue Drive
Suite 203
Bellevue, WA 98005
206/451-1984

Office of the Secretary of State
Legislative Bldg.
Olympia, WA 98504
206/753-7121

Washington
Public Disclosure Commission
403 Evergreen Plaza Building
Olympia, WA 98504
206/753-1111

West Virginia

West Virginia Democratic Headquarters
107 Pennsylvania Avenue

P.O. Box 6067
Charleston, WV 25302
304/342-8121

Republican State Executive Committee of West Virginia
P.O. Box 1007, Suite 1108 Union Building
Charleston, WV 25324
304/344-3446

Office of the Secretary of State
State Capitol, W-157
Charleston, WV 25305
304/348-2112

Elections Division
Office of the Secretary of State
State Capitol, Rm. 157
Charleston, WV 25305
304/348-3000

Wisconsin
Wisconsin (Madison)
Hours: 8:00–4:45
1/800/362-3020
In-state only. Handles general complaints and inquiries.

Wisconsin Democratic Headquarters
126 South Franklin Street
Madison, WI 53703
608/255-5172

Republican Party of Wisconsin
P.O. Box 31
(303 East Wilson Street)
Madison, WI 53701
608/257-4765

Office of the Secretary of State
State Capitol, Room 13 W.
Madison, WI 53702
608/266-5801

State Elections Board
125 S. Webster Street
Madison, WI 53702
608/266-8005

Wyoming
Wyoming Democratic Headquarters
P.O. Box 1964
Casper, WY 82502
307/234-8862

Wyoming Republican State Committee
P.O. Box 241
Casper, WY 82602
307/234-9166

Office of the Secretary of State
Capitol Building
Cheyenne, WY 82002
307/777-7378

Elections Division
Office of the Secretary of State
Capitol Building, Room 106
Cheyenne, WY 82002
307/777-7378

Appendix B:
National and State
Political and Professional
Organizations

This appendix lists national and state organizations that will provide political and professional information. It is by no means comprehensive. We have included those organizations that might provide the most information for health professionals new to political activity, that could make referrals to other helpful organizations, and that could be potential members of a network or coalition. As you increase your political activity, you will, of course, add to this list.

National Organizations

American Civil Liberties Union
22 E. 40th Street
New York, NY 10016
This organization defends individual rights granted by the U.S. Constitution, suits and amicus curiae briefs on behalf of persons, even when the right being defended is not popular.

American Nurses' Association, Inc.
N-CAP
1030 15th St., N.W.
Washington, DC 20005

Political action arm of the American Nurses Association. Focuses on education about political activities and fund raising to support candidates who have demonstrated support for nursing and health care. Contact N-CAP for state N-PAC.

Common Cause
2030 M. St. N.W.
Washington, DC 20036
(202) 833-1200
This organization has been active in government reform. Conducts studies for statistical information. Call for number of local office nearest you.

League of Women Voters
1730 M. St. N.W.
Washington, DC 20005
(202) 296-1770
Provides information to *all* voters. Sponsors programs, discussions, debates that clarify issues and candidates' views. Call national organization or refer to telephone book for state organization nearest you.

The National League for Nursing
10 Columbus Circle
New York, NY 10019
(212) 582-1022
Membership is open to nurses, other healthcare professionals, and members of the public interested in nursing. Publishes a number of resources including those on political activity.

National Women's Political Caucus
1411 K St., N.W., Suite 1110
Washington, DC 20005
(202) 347-4456
Focuses efforts on increasing the number of women in elected office, including judgeships.

Federation of Specialty Nursing Organizations
P.O. Box 23836
L'Enfant Playn, S.W.
Washington, DC 20026
Focuses on communication between nurse-specialty organizations and the American Nurses Association and on developing coalitions to work at the state level. The following organizations are members. For addresses and telephone numbers, refer to the following list of national health organizations:

> American Association of Critical-Care Nurses
> American Association of Nephrology Nurses and Technicians
> American Association of Nurse Anesthetists
> American Association of Occupational Health Nurses, Inc.
> American College of Nurse Midwives
> American Nurses Association
> American Public Health Association
> American Urological Association Allied
> The Association of Operating Room Nurses, Inc.
> Association of Practitioners in Infection Control
> Association of Rehabilitation Nurses
> Emergency Department Nurses' Association
> International Association for Enterostomal Therapy
> National Association of Pediatric Nurses Associates and Practitioners
> National Intravenous Therapy Association, Inc.
> National Nurses' Society of Alcoholism
> The Nurses's Association of the American College of Obstetricians and Gynecologists
> Oncology Nursing Society
> Orthopedic Nurses, Inc.

National Professional Organizations

Academy of Pharmacy Practice
c/o American Pharmaceutical Association

2215 Constitution Ave., N.W.
Washington, DC 20037
(202) 628-4410

American Academy of Ambulatory Nursing Administration
N. Woodbury Rd., Box 56
Pitman, NJ 08071
(609) 582-9617

American Academy of Nursing
2420 Pershing Rd.
Kansas City, MO 64108
(816) 474-5720

American Assembly for Men in Nursing
c/o College of Nursing
Rush University
600 S. Paulina, 474-H
Chicago, IL 60612
(312) 942-7117

American Association of Critical Care Nurses
1 Civic Plaza
Newport Beach, CA 92660
(714) 644-9310

American Association of Colleges of Nursing
11 Dupont Circle N.W., Suite 430
Washington, DC 20036
(202) 332-1917

American Association of Nephrology Nurses and Technicians
2 Talcott Rd., Suite B
Park Ridge, IL 60008

American Association of Neuroscience Nurses
22 S. Washington St., #203

Park Ridge, IL 60068
(312) 823-9850

American Association of Neurosurgical Nurses
625 N. Michigan Ave.
Suite 1519
Chicago, IL 60611

American Association of Nurse Anesthetists
216 W. Higgins Road
Park Ridge, IL 60068
(312) 692-7050

American Association of Occupational Health Nurses, Inc.
3500 Piedont Road, N.E.
Atlanta, GA 30305
(404) 262-1162

American College Health Association
152 Rollings Ave., Suite 208
Rockville, MD 20852
(301) 468-6868

American College of Health Care Administrators
P.O. Box 5890
4650 East-West Hwy.
Bethesda, MD 20814
(301) 652-8384

American College of Nurse-Midwives
1522 K St., N.W., Suite 1120
Washington, DC 20005
(202) 347-5445

American Dental Hygenists Association
444 N. Michigan Ave.
Chicago, IL 60611
(312) 440-8900

American Dietetic Association
430 N. Michigan Ave.
Chicago, IL 60611
(312) 280-5000

American Health Care Association
1200 15th St., N.W.
Washington, DC 20005
(202) 833-2050

American Indian/Alaska Native Nurses Association
P.O. 3908
Lawrence, KS 66044
(913) 749-4335

American Institute of Nutrition
9650 Rockville Pike
Bethesda, MD 20814
(301) 530-7050

American Nurses Association
2420 Pershing Road
Kansas City, MO 64108
(816) 474-5720

American Occupational Therapy Association
1383 Piccard Drive Suite 301
Rockville, MD 20850
(301) 948-9626

American Pharmaceutical Association
2215 Constitution Ave., N.W.
Washington, DC 20037
(202) 628-4410

American Physical Therapy Association
1156 15th Street, N.W.

Washington, DC 20005
(202) 466-2070

American Public Health Association
1015 15th St., N.W.
Washington, DC 20005
(202) 789-5600

American School Health Association
P.O. Box 708
1521 S. Water Street
Kent, OH 44240
(216) 678-1601

American Society for Medical Technology
330 Meadowfern Drive
Houston, TX 77067
(713) 893-7072

American Society for Nursing Service Administrators
AHA Bldg.
840 N. Lake Shore Dr.
Chicago, IL 60611
(312) 280-6410

American Society for Parenteral and Enteral Nutrition
1025 Vermont Ave., Suite 810
Washington, DC 20005
(202) 638-5881

American Society of Consultant Pharmacists
2300 Ninth St., S., Suite 503
Arlington, VA 22204
(703) 920-8492

American Society of Plastic and Reconstructive Surgical Nurses
23341 N. Milwaukee Ave.

Half Day, IL 60069
(312) 634-1405

American Society of Post-anesthesia Nurses
P.O. Box 11083
Richmond, VA 23230
(804) 359-3557

American Urological Association Allied
21510 S. Main St.
Carson, CA 90745

Association for Advancement of Health Education
1900 Association Drive
Reston, VA 22091
(703) 476-3440

Association of Operating Room Nurses, Inc. (The)
10170 E. Mississippi Ave.
Denver, CO 80231

Association of Pediatric Oncology Nurses
c/o Lorraine Bivalec
Pediatric Oncology
Pacific Medical Center
P.O. Box 7999
San Francisco, CA 94120
(415) 563-8777

Association of Practitioners in Infection Control
P.O. Box 546
Palatine, IL 60067

Association of Rehabilitation Nurses
2506 Gross Point Road
Evanston, IL 60201
(312) 475-7530

Association of State and Territorial Directors of Nursing
c/o Geraldine Price
Division of Nursing
Ohio Dep. of Health
P.O. Box 118
Columbus, OH 43216
(614) 466-2205

Dermatology Nurses Association
Box 56, N. Woodbury Rd.
Pitman, NJ 08071
(609) 582-1915

Emergency Department Nurses Association
666 N. Lakeshore Dr.
Chicago, IL 60611
(312) 649-0297

International Association for Enterostomal Therapy
505 N. Tustin Ave., Suite 219
Santa Ana, CA 92705

National Association for Practical Nurse Education and Service
254 W. 31st St.
New York, NY 10001
(212) 736-4540

National Association of Hispanic Nurses
115 Magnolia Dr.
San Antonio, TX 78212
(512) 733-7460

National Association of Nurse Recruiters
Box 56, N. Woodbury Rd.
Pitman, NJ 08071
(609) 582-1915

National Association of Orthopaedic Nurses
Box 56, N. Woodbury Rd.
Pitman, NJ 08071
(609) 582-0111

National Association of Pediatric Nurse Associates and Practitioners
Box 56
N. Woodbury Road
Pitman, NJ 08071
(609) 589-5077

National Association of Physician Nurses
3837 Plaza Dr.
Fairfax, VA 22030
(703) 273-6262

National Association of Quality Assurance Professionals
1800 Pickwick Ave.
Glenview, IL 60025
(312) 724-7700

National Association of School Nurses
7395 S. Krameria St.
Englewood, CO 80112
(303) 850-9033

National Black Nurses Association
P.O. Box 18358
Boston, MA 02118
(617) 266-9703

National Board of Pediatric Nurse Practitioners and Associates
414 Hungerford Dr., Suite 310
Rockville, MD 20850
(301) 340-8213

National Federation of Licensed Practical Nurses
P.O. Box 11038
214 S. Driver Street
Durham, NC 27703
(919) 596-9609

National Flight Nurse Association
c/o Roy Evans
Life Flight Southern California
P.O. Box 1420
Long Beach, CA 90801
(213) 426-0378

National Intravenous Therapy Association, Inc.
850 Third Ave, 11th Floor
New York, NY 10022

National League for Nursing
10 Columbus Circle
New York, NY 10019
(212) 582-1022

National Licensed Practical Nurses Educational Foundation
P.O. Box 11038
Durham, NC 27703
(919) 596-9609

National Nurses Society on Addictions
2506 Gross Point Rd.
Evanston, IL 60201
(312) 475-7530

National Nurses Society on Alcoholism
733 Third Ave.
New York, NY 10017

National Registry of Emergency Medical Technicians
P.O. Box 29233
Columbus, OH 43229
(614) 888-4484

National Student Nurses' Association
10 Columbus Circle
New York, NY 10019
(212) 581-2211

Nurses Association of the American College of Obstetricians and
  Gynecologists
600 Maryland Ave., S.W., Suite 200
Washington, DC 20024
(202) 638-0026

Nurses Organization of the Veterans Administration
23341 Milwaukee Ave.
Half Day, IL 60069
(312) 634-1412

Oncology Nursing Society
701 Washington Rd.
Pittsburg, PA 15228

Orthopedic Nurses, Inc.
3165 E. Shadowlaw
Atlanta, GA 30305

Otorhinolarynogology and Head/Neck Nurses
3893 E. Market St.
Warren, OH 44484
(216) 856-4000

Society for Public Health Education, Inc.
703 Market Street, Suite 535
San Francisco, CA 94103
(216) 678-1601

State Professional Organizations

The following organizations are associated with the American Nurses' Association, Inc. To obtain the name, address, and telephone of the state president or executive director of other state healthcare organizations, call the national organization.

Alabama
Alabama State Nurses' Association
360 North Hull Street
Montgomery, AL 36104
(205) 262-8321

Alaska
Alaska Nurses Association
237 East Third Avenue
Anchorage, AK 99501
(907) 274-0827

Arizona
Arizona Nurses' Association
4525 North 12th Street
Phoenix, AZ 85014
(602) 277-4401

Arkansas
Arkansas State Nurses' Association
117 South Cedar Street
Little Rock, AR 72205
(501) 664-5853

California
California Nurses Association
1855 Folsom Street, Room 670
San Francisco, CA 94103
(415) 864-4141

Colorado
Colorado Nurses' Association
5453 East Evans Place
Denver, CO 80222
(303) 757-7484

Connecticut
Connecticut Nurses' Association
1 Prestige Drive
Meriden, CT 06450
(203) 238-1208

Delaware
Delaware Nurses' Association
111 East 42nd Street
Wilmington, DE 19802
(302) 764-5762

District of Columbia
District of Columbia Nurses' Association, Inc.
5100 Wisconsin Ave., N.W., Suite 306
Washington, DC 20016
(202) 244-2705

Florida
Florida Nurses Association
P.O. Box 6985
1235 East Concord Street
Orlando, FL 32803
(Packages or bulk mailings to 1235 E. Concord)
(305) 896-3261

Georgia
Georgia Nurses Association, Inc.
1362 West Peachtree Street, N.W.
Atlanta, GA 30309
(404) 876-4624

Hawaii
Hawaii Nurses Association
677 Ala Moana Boulevard, Suite 607
Honolulu, HI 96813
(808) 531-1628

Idaho
Idaho Nurses Association
1134 North Orchard, Suite 8
Boise, ID 83706
(208) 377-0226

Illinois
Illinois Nurses' Association
20 North Wacker Drive, Suite 2520
Chicago, IL 60606
(312) 236-9708

Indiana
Indiana State Nurses' Association
2915 North High School Road
Indianapolis, IN 46224
(317) 299-4575/4576

Iowa
Iowa Nurses' Association
Shops Building, Room 215
Des Moines, IA 50309
(515) 282-9169

Kansas
Kansas State Nurses' Association
820 Quincy Street
Topeka, KS 66612
(913) 233-8638

Kentucky
Kentucky Nurses Association
P.O. Box 8342
Louisville, KY 40208-0342
(502) 637-2546/2547

Louisiana
Louisiana State Nurses Association
712 Transcontinental Drive
Metairie, LA 70001
(504) 889-1030

Maine
Maine State Nurses' Association
P.O. Box 2240
Augusta, ME 04330
(207) 622-1057

Maryland
Maryland Nurses Association, Inc.
5820 Southwestern Boulevard
Baltimore, MD 21227
(301) 242-7300

Massachusetts
Massachusetts Nurses Association
376 Boylson Street
Boston, MA 02116
(617) 482-5465

Michigan
Michigan Nurses Association
120 Spartan Avenue
East Lansing, MI 48823
(517) 337-1653

Minnesota
Minnesota Nurses Association
Griggs-Midway Building, Suite 152
1821 University Avenue
St. Paul, MN 55104
(612) 646-4807

Mississippi
Mississippi Nurses' Association
135 Bounds Street, Suite 100
Jackson, MS 39206
(601) 982-9182

Missouri
Missouri Nurses Association
206 East Dunklin Street, Box 325
Jefferson City, MO 65101
(314) 636-4623

Montana
Montana Nurses' Association
2001 Eleventh Avenue
P.O. Box 5718
Helena, MT 59601
(406) 442-6710

Nebraska
Nebraska Nurses' Association
941 "O" Street, Suite 707-711
Lincoln, NE 68508
(402) 475-3859

Nevada
Nevada Nurses' Association
3660 Baker Lane
Reno, NV 89509
(702) 825-3555

New Hampshire
New Hampshire Nurses' Association
48 West Street
Concord, NH 03301
(603) 225-3783

New Jersey
New Jersey State Nurses Association
320 West State Street
Trenton, NJ 08618
(609) 392-4884

New Mexico
New Mexico Nurses' Association
525 San Pedro, N.E., Suite 100
Albuquerque, NM 87108
(505) 268-7744

New York
New York State Nurses Association
2113 Western Avenue
Guilderland, NY 12084
(518) 456-5371

North Carolina
North Carolina Nurses Association
Box 12025
103 Enterprise Street
Raleigh, NC 27605
(919) 821-4250

North Dakota
North Dakota State Nurses Association
Green Tree Square
212 North Fourth Street
Bismarck, ND 58501
(701) 223-1385

Ohio
Ohio Nurses Association
P.O. Box 13169
4000 East Main Street
Columbus, OH 43213
(614) 237-5414

Oklahoma
Oklahoma Nurses Association
Suite A
6414 North Santa Fe
Oklahoma City, OK 73116
(405) 840-3476

Oregon
Oregon Nurses Association, Inc.
Scholls West, Suite 103
9730 S.W. Cascade Boulevard
Tigard, OR 97223
(503) 620-7474

Pennsylvania
Pennsylvania Nurses Association
P.O. Box 8525
2515 North Front Street
Harrisburg, PA 17105-8525
(Packages or bulk mailings to 2515 North Front Street)
(717) 234-7935

Rhode Island
Rhode Island State Nurses' Association
345 Blackstone Boulevard
Hall Building South
Providence, RI 02906
(401) 421-9703

South Carolina
South Carolina Nurses' Association
1821 Gadsden Street
Columbia, SC 29201
(803) 252-4781

South Dakota
South Dakota Nurses' Association, Inc.
1505 South Minnesota, Suite #6
Sioux Falls, SD 57105
(605) 338-1401

Tennessee
Tennessee Nurses' Association
1720 West End Building, Suite 400
Nashville, TN 37203
(615) 329-2511

Texas
Texas Nurses Association
314 Highland Mall Boulevard, Suite 504
Austin, TX 78752
(512) 452-0645

Utah
Utah Nurses' Association
1058 East 900 South
Salt Lake City, UT 84105
(801) 322-3439/3430

Vermont
Vermont State Nurses Association, Inc.
500 Dorset Street
South Burlington, VT 05401
(802) 864-9390

Virginia
Virginia Nurses' Association
1311 High Point Avenue
Richmond, VA 23230
(804) 353-7311

Washington
Washington State Nurses Association
2615 Fourth Avenue, Suite 380
4th and Vine Building
Seattle, WA 98121
(206) 622-3613

West Virginia
West Virginia Nurses' Association, Inc.
Union Building, Suite 511
723 Kanawha Boulevard, East
Charleston, WV 25301
(304) 342-7978

Wisconsin
Wisconsin Nurses Association, Inc.
206 East Olin Avenue
Madison, WI 53713
(608) 251-1462

Wyoming
Wyoming Nurses' Association
Majestic Building, Room 305
1603 Capitol Avenue
Cheyenne, WY 82001
(307) 635-3955

Index